Integrating Spirituality and Occupational Therapy Treatment

Integrating Spirituality and Occupational Therapy Treatment

A Practical Guide

Dr. Laura Ayres Hayth, SsD, OTR/L, CHC

ISBN: 1511889314
ISBN 13: 9781511889315
Library of Congress Control Number: 2015906941
CreateSpace Independent Publishing Platform
North Charleston, South Carolina

Cover: Original watercolor art by Laura Hayth
Author photo and photo of original art by
Glenn Schafer Photography, www.GlennSchafer.com
Disclaimer: Patient initials in the vignette chapters were changed to protect identities.

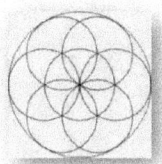

This book is dedicated to my family and friends who are the inherent Divine orchestra of my spiritual journey and symphony, and to all the health-care professionals who have the power to transform themselves and the world, one person at a time, to the sacred roots and wings of spiritual healing in mind, body and spirit.

CONTENTS

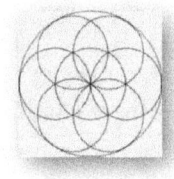

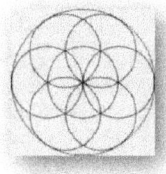

The energy of the mind is the essence of life...

~ARISTOTLE

1

A Greater Purpose:
Path of Sacred Action

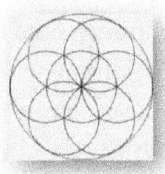

There is a vitality, a life force, an energy, a quickening, that is translated through you into action, and because there is only one of you in all time, this expression is unique.

~Martha Graham

Occupational therapy and a spirituality-based approach to therapeutic intervention are naturally intertwined. Based on a person's culture, coping skills, and lifestyle, self-efficacy and self-determination give one a sense of control in life through occupation. Occupation means any *meaningful* activity. We are all inherently and fundamentally connected whether we believe that or not. How a person perceives his or her personal sacred or awe-inspiring reverence, in personal *connection* to the Universe, Spirit, Source, the Divine, Mystery, Truth, Higher Power, the Earth, or the God of his or her understanding or merely living a moral and just life with meaning and purpose—and to the natural environment, friends, family, and community—is the foundation of self-efficacy and a sense of the "sacred higher self."

The restoration of this fundamental core belief system of faith and intricate meaningful and sacred *connection*, if disrupted in one's awareness and perception of awareness—through disability, injury, pain, mental illness, and fear of death or the unknown—is a vital component of occupational therapy intervention. The sense of *dis-connectivity,* or *separation,* affects self-efficacy, self-esteem, and self-healing.

There is a paradigm shift occurring in the world's perception of true wellness that emphasizes the mind–body–spirit connection. Therapeutic treatment that includes strategies to empower patients, residents, and clients to reconnect to joy and peace through prayer, meditation, guided imagery, or other positive therapeutic activities in order to recognize and reconnect to their awareness of the sacred self are essential to physical, mental, and spiritual healing. Reconnection of spiritual awareness is inherently vital to successful therapeutic outcomes in returning to meaningful activity in any and all occupational therapy health-care settings.

Occupational Therapy

The Occupational Therapy Practice Framework (AOTA 2014b) defines occupational therapy as

> the therapeutic use of everyday life activities (occupations) with individuals or groups for the purpose of enhancing or enabling participation in roles, habits, and routines in home, school, workplace, community, and other settings. Occupational therapy practitioners use their knowledge of the transactional relationship among the person, his or her engagement in valuable occupations, and the context to design occupation-based intervention plans that facilitate change or growth in client factors (body functions, body structures, values, beliefs, and spirituality) and skills (motor, process, and social interaction) needed for successful participation. Occupational therapy practitioners are concerned with the end result of participation and thus enable engagement through adaptations and modifications to the environment or objects within the environment when needed. Occupational therapy services are provided for habilitation, rehabilitation, and promotion

of health and wellness for clients with disability- and non-disability-related needs. These services include acquisition and preservation of occupational identity for those who have or at risk for developing illness, injury, disease, disorder, condition, impairment, disability, activity limitation or participation restrictions. (p. S1)

Occupational Therapists (OTs) and Certified Occupational Therapy Assistants (COTAs) help people of all ages across the life span to restore, remediate, or adapt a patient's ability to participate in bathing, dressing, home management, school, work, play, and socialization—all within the context of a patient's habits, culture, values, beliefs, and spirituality (Hooper and Wood 2014).

Hooper and Wood (2014, 38) stated:

A core philosophical assumption of the profession, therefore, is that by virtue of our biological endowment, people of all ages and abilities require occupations to grow, and thrive; in pursuing occupation, humans express the totality of their being, a mind-body-spirit union. Because human existence could not otherwise be, humankind is, in essence, occupational by nature.

Practitioners (OTs and COTAs collectively) can realize a greater purpose by changing and setting the therapeutic intentions to a *path of sacred action*. Practitioners are in a unique position to be of deep value to their patients, residents, or clients, first, by understanding how to bring their whole and centered self to the table of providing therapy in a way that goes beyond basic rapport—to deep listening, to sacred connection, and to a path of sacred action with the people they serve. They need to be anchored and aligned in their own connection and in their own sacred spiritual belief system. To promote the sacred in others, one must be open and accepting of every individual path to Spirit in its many forms. Practitioners need a commitment to be unbiased and to honor all authentic spiritual, religious, and nonreligious paths to Truth, regardless of their own personal belief system.

Second, practitioners need a greater understanding of the nature of spirituality, how spirituality affects health and wellness, and the difference between spirituality and religion. We are all connected. We are all pure energy with different levels of vibrational frequency. We are spiritual beings having a human experience. We all have inherent and integral value to the whole. We are all just *walking one another home.* When people lose sight of their core belief system—their spiritual connection, or their version of meaning and purpose—that perception of *disconnection* is directly related to *dis-ease.* Disconnection—or lack of awareness of the inherent connection infinitely present—and disease in mind, body, or spirit is a root cause and effect. The lack of awareness and sense of disconnection lowers our vibration frequency. The perceived disconnection that often happens during a health crisis also leads to fear—fear of outcomes, fear of the unknown, and fear of dying or being forgotten—which greatly inhibits one's ability to naturally self-heal. Signs of disconnection include feelings of helplessness, hopelessness, and isolation—feeling completely alone in the world. Reconnecting to one's personal core belief systems and finding and remembering the deep and sacred roots of connection enables the sacred wings of healing mentally, physically, and spiritually by literally restoring our vibrational frequency to a state of balance, and is the basis of empowerment toward self-efficacy, deep acceptance, and handling the reality of what is. We offer occupational therapy services to give sacred roots and wings to the people we serve: roots of Spiritual reconnection in order to have the wings for Spiritual healing in mind, body, and spirit. A primary focus of roots and wings is thus enabling all other therapy strategies to be successful.

Third, practitioners need a basic understanding of the tools, available resources, and therapeutic strategies that can be utilized for assisting others in spiritual reconnection and how to inspire and empower people to reconnect to the truth of their understanding. There are many adjunct therapeutic activities that can be applied to enable individuals to reconnect and remember who they are as spiritual beings. Practitioners can be the catalyst for going beyond just treating patients and sending them home. We have the opportunity to change people's lives in mind, body, and spirit by moving from treating to caring (Gawande 2014) and bringing a mind-set of sacred action to caring for every patient, resident, or client. Ultimately, practitioners can help people to walk in reverence to their connection and inspire vibrational increase for self-healing emotionally, physically, and spiritually. Sharing our stories of deep connection bridges the humanity in all of us.

2

Religion and Spirituality

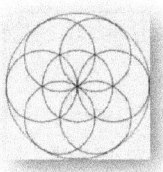

How much longer will you go on letting your energy sleep? How much longer are you going to stay oblivious of the immensity of yourself?

~BHAGWAN SHREE RAJNEESH

Including spirituality in occupational therapy treatment is part of the Occupational Therapy Practice Act and is within our scope of practice; however, there is minimal understanding of what that means or how to go about it. Many OTs acknowledge that spirituality may be included in the plan of care and therapeutic approach to patient care; however, spirituality as a therapeutic intervention has not been adequately researched and has not been effectively taught in the occupational therapy educational system. Some OTs and COTAs believe that they have to understand a patient's religion and are not comfortable with that aspect and defer to religious professionals, omitting an opportunity to facilitate a vital aspect of occupational therapy treatment that would be highly beneficial to patients.

Spirituality goes beyond a patient's religion, focusing more universally and metaphysically on the patient's sacred *individual* connection to Spirit that is thought to be distinctly meaningful. A sense of spiritual connection and

reconnection will often be the motivating factor for him or her to participate in activities that are personally and individually meaningful, purposeful,
valuable, and significant. Spirituality *is* connection.

Even people who do not believe in a higher power usually have a belief
system that contains a personal moral code of conduct that they live by,
which defines meaning to them that leads to living their higher self, creating
a personal perception of the sacred or significant in living. Therefore, if one
lives by a personal moral code, one is creating purpose and meaning while
striving for the sacred higher self; that is living a spiritual life, whether one
calls it that or not. Whether one believes in God, Source, the Divine, the
All There Is, the Universe, or nothing, this connection is universal and vital
even if we are not aware of it. Marianne Williamson, an American spiritual
teacher, author, and lecturer says, "Everyone is on a spiritual path. Most
people just don't know it." (theartofancientwisdom.com 4.21.14) A person's
sense of connection, if not to Spirit, but to the earth and to a sense of shared
community, is also Spirituality.

We are all *one*. As a deeply connected living, breathing world and cosmic
community, we all have an inherent value to the whole. We bring our unique
gifts to share with the world, and we make a difference just by being. The
strength of our connection to a higher self or higher power is what gets us
through adversity *and* success. Ultimately, this connection is how we increase
our vibration in order to heal ourselves mentally, physically, and spiritually.
We are all part of this sacred connection; whether we perceive our sacred
connection through a customary spiritual lens or through a sacred earth community as our higher-self lens, the sense of connection is vital to our health in
mind, body, and spirit.

Practitioners need to understand the key role they have that can be beneficial to helping patients uncover the false sense of separation, which often
occurs through illness, disease, or fear. This strategy requires deep listening.
Per the contemplativemind.org website, deep listening is a way of hearing in
which we are fully present with what is happening in the moment. Truly connecting to patients, residents, or clients requires one to practice compassion
and develop deep listening skills.

OTs have the unique opportunity to teach patients coping skills that foster this sacred connection. Strategies promoting a healing "attitude of gratitude," leading to a grateful heart, and meditation activities that promote the practice of being present in the moment through mindfulness are examples of ways to empower a patient to reconnect to their revered and inherent universal value to the whole. Promoting this connection encourages coping skills to deal with the challenges of chronic pain, chronic mental illness, fear of death or the unknown, or physical disability through that reconnection and ultimately toward self-healing. Nurturing the sacred in others is also beneficial to the therapist's own personal growth and development of his or her personal higher self.

Religion

The Universal Mystery is a great equalizer across all world cultures and throughout all time. We all come face-to-face with the unknown and the unknowable. There are many vastly unique religions in the world. Religion is a major social institution, and each a particular group or system of faith and worship, organized in a specific collection of beliefs, cultural systems, and worldviews. Practices and rituals are generally agreed upon and related to by the group in a certain way toward humankind within a context of meaning for each group.

Religious concepts, often described as structured, symbolic, and ritualistic, are formally or informally taught, and are frequently handed down from generation to generation within a culture. At times, religion can be noninclusive in that some segments believe they have the right path to the Divine and often judge or hold in contempt those who do not believe exactly the way they do. This is a group-think interpretation of the teachings that define someone else's experiences to be the truth.

A person can be religious or spiritual or both. Some religious people seem to just follow the rules as set forth by their particular brand of religion with no real personal connection to the God path of their choice. Other religious people feel very spiritual and have a strong personal connection to the God of their understanding. Even an agnostic or atheist—for example, a person growing up in a nonreligious family who was encouraged to have fundamental compassion for others, participate in community volunteerism, have a high moral code to live by, and have purpose and meaning—is actually living a spiritual life.

There are signs of change in the modern world, however, due to a paradigm shift in global spiritual thinking. It seems the world wants change in the form of love and acceptance. Some traditional churches are seeing a decline in attendance due to a general dissatisfaction in leadership and a sense of deep disconnect in organized religion. The world wants more—more meaning, more belonging, more inclusion, and a need to feel part of the whole. New-thought spiritual philosophy is filling that void. Some significant changes are happening right now in the traditional religions as well.

"Religion is another example of social contract disengagement" (Brown 2012, 176). Disengagement occurs when leaders do not live by the same values that they preach, and turn faith into compliance and consequences. "Spiritual connection and engagement is not built on compliance; it's the product of love, belonging, and vulnerability" (Brown 2012, 177).

We have evidence of a paradigm shift occurring in action in recent world events. In Catholicism, for example, Pope Francis has encouragingly made concerted efforts to demonstrate more tolerance and a tone of inclusivity in his actions and words, which have been very well received throughout the world by Catholics and non-Catholics alike, and has made him a very popular pope. He has been brave in voicing honest criticism of the Church has embraced people of other faiths and those with no faith at all, and has encouraged open debate and conversations. This is called the "Francis effect." However, not all Catholics are satisfied with the time it is taking to effect real change, and that the much-needed shifts may not even happen during Francis's papacy (Kuruvilla 2015).

In addition, the 126-year-old Central Conference of American Rabbis welcomed its first openly gay president, Rabbi Denise Eger, on March 16, 2015. She has also been a member of its board of trustees for four years and is the founding rabbi of the lesbian, gay, bisexual, and transgender (LGBT) community–friendly Los Angeles synagogue Kol Ami. She is a human rights activist and shares her interpretations of the Torah on her blog. "Reform Judaism and Reform rabbis have long been on the forefront of civil rights," and the process of re-inspiration is also one of modernization as reform communities "move proudly and faithfully into the twenty-first century," according to Rabbi Eger (Bloomberg, 3.13.15, huffingtonpost.com). A new prayer book released by the reform movement reflects this shift with LGBT-friendly language and gender inclusivity (Blumberg 2015).

Spirituality

"Spirituality is the aspect of humanity that refers to the way individuals seek and express meaning and purpose and the way they experience their connectedness to the moment, to self, to others, to nature, and to the significant or sacred" (Puchalski, Ferrell, Virani, Otis-Green, Baird, Bull, Chochinov, Handzo, Nelson-Becker, Prince-Paul, Pugliese, and Sulmasy, 2009, 887).

Spirituality is frequently described as the experience of having one's *own* personal relationship to the sacred and is largely inclusive and accepting of other points of view. Spirituality, then, is the thread in the tapestry of all truths that exists in all religions. Spirituality is the key to living greatly and dying gracefully.

Viktor Frankl, a Jewish psychiatrist imprisoned by the Nazis, once said, "Man is ready and willing to shoulder any suffering as soon and as long as he can see meaning in it." Frankl used his cruel and vicious experience in the concentration camps to gain insight into how people did or did not survive. Survival wasn't based on age or bodily strength, but rather, "on the strength derived from purpose, and discovering the meaning in one's life and experience" (Dalai Lama and Cutler 1998, 199). Frankl has taught us how to live, out of the devastation of this experience.

Wayne Dyer, an internationally renowned author and speaker in the fields of self-development and spiritual growth, wrote a wonderful book on interpreting the wisdom of Lao-tzu in the *Tao Te Ching* (a book of Chinese wisdom poetry written 2,500 years ago) for the modern world. Based on this great work, Dyer teaches that we live in a world aligned with nature. Find ways to live and enjoy the Mystery. Let go of naming and labeling everything as good or bad and focus on oneness and acceptance. There is no way to happiness: happiness is the way, and we have to trust the process (Dyer 2007).

Joseph Campbell, an American mythologist, writer, and lecturer best known for his work in comparative mythology and comparative religion, said the modern hero is the modern individual "who dares to heed the call and seek the mansion of that presence with whom it is our whole destiny to be atoned, cannot, indeed must not, wait for his community to cast off its slough of pride, fear, rationalized avarice, and sanctified misunderstanding" (Campbell, 1949, 391). Humans must rediscover the mystery and regain "the focal point of human wonder" (Campbell 1949, 391).

Religions are unique and touch on spirituality in different ways. There are similar insights on spirituality in many diverse philosophies, religions, teachings, and traditions. Looking at these diverse insights helps to see the golden thread that connects us all. From buddahgroove.com, insights below are part of the golden thread in the tapestry of all truths:

Jesus: In the Gospel of Thomas, "that which you seek is already here, but you do not recognize it."

Buddha: No one saves us but ourselves. No one can and no one may. We ourselves must walk the path.

Lao-tzu: Do you have the patience to wait until your mud settles and the water is clear?

Hinduism: Go within yourself, and what you achieve there will overshadow your imperfections. (Sri Chinmoy)

Baha'i: With the human soul, there is no decline. Its only movement is toward perfection; growth and progress alone constitute the motion of the soul.

Sufism: If you wish to find what you are looking for, remove that which hides your heart. (Kabir)

Zen Philosophy: With the sound of water falling into a stone bowl, suddenly the dust of your mind has been washed away. (Sen-No-Rikyu)

Judaism: Let your heart become ever more humble so that you may give yourself equally to all. Then you will be capable of meditating. (Isaac of Acco)

Catholicism: If a man wishes to be sure of the road he treads on, he must close his eyes and walk in the dark. (St. John of the Cross)

Classical Philosophy: Look well into thyself; there is a source of strength, which will always spring up if thou wilt always look. (Marcus Aurelius)

"The search for deeper existence is a common in many of our lives. In our seeking, words of wisdom may help us navigate the journey within" (Buddhagroove.com 2015). New Thought spirituality and philosophy is compatible with many religious teachings and is being embraced by many people.

3

History of New Thought/Spirituality

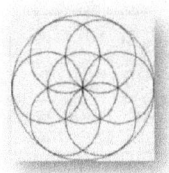

Self-realization means that we have been consciously connected
with our source of being. Once we have made this connection,
then nothing can go wrong...

~SWAMI PARAMANANDA

Understanding the history of New Thought evolution is a vital key for the practitioner to fully grasp the concepts of the philosophy and the principles that apply to helping patients in reconnecting to their spiritual connection: to the God of their understanding or to the concept of higher self and of being an inherent part of the whole.

There is a spiritual revolution going on in the world, a growing trend of spiritually independent people who do not want to confine their path to any institution. Some would call it a revolt against the confines of organized religion. However, this philosophy is a companion and a complementary strategic way to increase and realize a personal relationship with Spirit or find meaning in the "knowing" that we are part of the whole within a chosen religious construct or independent beliefs. The New Thought revolution relates spirituality to metaphysics. Modern New Thought spiritual leader and writer Eckhart Tolle defines spirituality as the arising new consciousness, drawing on the ancient masters and writings such as Buddha; Lao-tzu; the *Tao Te Ching*; Jesus, and the Bible, the book sacred to Christians containing the New Testament and the Old Testament, which is sacred to Jews; the Bhagavad Gita, a book of Hindu scriptures; and many other ancient teachings. In his book *A New Earth: Awakening to Your Life's Purpose,* Tolle explains how these teachings all had different names for this new consciousness or transformation: enlightenment, salvation, end of suffering, and awakening. These masters spoke to their masses about sin, suffering, and delusion (Tolle 2005, 14).

The New Thought movement in the nineteenth and twentieth centuries was founded on world religions and teachings. The prominent thinkers, spiritual leaders, and writers of the time were Ralph Waldo Emerson, Henry David Thoreau, Emma Curtis Hopkins, Ernest Holmes, Thomas Troward, Myrtle and Charles Fillmore, Emmet Fox, and Joseph Campbell, to name a few. They communicated through books, magazines, and articles, and later in the twentieth century, on television through PBS specials, which included Joseph Campbell interviews. Books of this era by these authors are considered classics.

Ralph Waldo Emerson was a philosopher, poet, journalist, and transcendentalist in the nineteenth century. He graduated from Harvard School of Divinity and was licensed and ordained as a minister in the Unitarian Church in 1829. He wrote on the nature of spiritual experience and ethical living. He cofounded the literary magazine *The Dial,* and his best-known essays include "Self Reliance," "Friendship," and "Experience." He strongly influenced his literary group, known as the American Transcendentalists, with the key belief that God was not remote or unknowable; that each individual could transcend the physical world of the senses into deeper spiritual experience through free will and intuition; and that one only had to look within one's own soul to find God through feeling one's own connection to nature. He is well known as the "Sage of Concord" (Massachusetts). His ideas and belief system were strong influences on the work of his protégé Henry David Thoreau and his contemporary Walt Whitman (http://www.transcendentalism-legacy-tamu-edu/ authors/emerson).

Judge Thomas Troward was an English author whose works were a powerful influence on the New Thought movement and mystic Christianity. His works strongly influenced Holmes and later New Thought teachers.

After he retired in 1896, he set out to apply logic and a judicial weighing of evidence in the study of matters of Spirit and matter, and cause and effect. In the Edinburgh Lectures on Mental Science in 1904, Troward explained that everything is energy, and despite outward appearances, what seems to be solid matter is actually energy flowing at a lower vibration. Everything in the universe is energy in vibration at different degrees of intelligence. In addition, Troward succinctly explained the Law of Mind: that the universal Mind is the Divine Mind and agrees with everything we think through the subconscious mind—the subjective mind—directly connected to Spirit. Spirit is thought. The subconscious mind holds deep-seated beliefs that are subjective, compelled by subjective nature to accept and create without discernment. Subjective law is impersonal. Because we have free will, Spirit agrees with everything we think. Troward eloquently portrayed the link between thought and manifestation of reality. What a person puts his or her attention to expands. So if you dwell in negative thoughts, a doomsday focus will get you just that. Conversely, if you are a positive thinker with a positive focus in thought patterns and you guard your thoughts, then you foster a positive reality (Troward, 1904).

Dr. Ernest Holmes, an American spiritual writer, teacher, and leader, was the founder of a spiritual movement known as Religious Science, a part of the greater New Thought movement whose spiritual philosophy is recognized also as the Science of Mind. He wrote many beloved metaphysical books and was the founder of *Science of Mind* magazine, which has been in circulation since 1927. In 1926 he wrote the book *The Science of Mind,* a seminal work and a teaching text still used worldwide and a reference source for Science of Mind philosophy. He founded the Institute of Religious Science, and the Church of Religious Science, which is now called United Centers for Spiritual Living. Religious Science is globally known, promoting universal truths and the ultimate Oneness of Universal Life.

Holmes's teachings promote a reawakening of each individual's awareness of his or her higher self, or his or her sacred connection to the All There Is. God is a universal presence existing in our own soul and operating in our own consciousness—not outside of the self to beg to, but already accessible through mind. "Holmes developed a universal philosophy and tools for spiritual living that profoundly resonate to this day. His work provides us with a personal spiritual path, and understanding of our relationship with the universe and a connected and joyful approach to daily living. Ernest Holmes's work is recognized today as one of the leading viewpoints in modern metaphysics and New Thought" (scienceofmind.com).

Holmes developed a style of prayer called affirmative prayer with a focus on the positive outcome rather than a negative situation. For example, the practitioner would encourage a patient to focus the prayer or positive thought on the desired state of perfect health, as if it already happened, rather than identifying the illness and then asking God to help eliminate it.

Joseph Campbell was an American mythologist, writer, educator, and lecturer in mythology and comparative religion in the twentieth century, strongly influenced by Carl Jung and best known for his phrase "following your bliss." He believed in the unity of humankind and the eternal source constantly pouring into this world. When asked about the meaning of life, he responded, "There is no meaning. We bring meaning to it." Campbell taught that we can choose to live in rapture, that it is not "out there" in some other place or person, and that we don't have to go somewhere, or have something or someone. "It is *here*, it is *here*, it is *here*. A shift in consciousness is all it takes" (Olson 1991, 10).

In the twenty-first century, however, New Thought philosophy is exponentially exploding through the information highway of the globally accessible Internet. Current modern-day masters, mystics, writers, and leaders include Eckhart Tolle, Deepak Chopra, Wayne Dyer, the Dalai Lama, Thich Nhat Hanh, Marianne Williamson, Pema Chodron, Michael Bernard Beckwith, Sri Amma and Sri Bhagavan, John Lennon, Maya Angelou, and Carolyn Myss, among others. Communication avenues include books, magazines, music, articles, Internet, social media, and television.

GaiamTV is an Internet-based television station dedicated to spiritual programming. Thanks to Oprah Winfrey and *Super Soul Sunday*, on Oprah Winfrey Network (OWN) television, the global awareness of New Thought metaphysical, philosophical principles is much more mainstream today. Per a Winfrey network press release: "The Emmy Award–winning series *Super Soul Sunday* delivers a thought-provoking, eye-opening, and inspiring block of programming designed to help viewers awaken to their best selves and discover a deeper connection to the world around them." Oprah states that the reason she started OWN was "to gather a global community of like-minded seekers" (Oprah.com).

Facebook and the Internet have revolutionized how people get information, and the metaphysical following is extremely prevalent. Modern-day masters, mystics, and writers all have Facebook pages with loyal followers. The pages are full of information, articles, healthy living strategies, and daily tips and reminders. In addition, other metaphysical pages have emerged. Each of these pages has a familiar undertone but vary in flavor to suit one's taste. A few examples of popular pages include the following:

- Spirit Science: The Science of Spirit, in the Spirit of Science, coming together to create something new
- The Renaissance Project: a nonprofit organization to unify physics and spirit science education with focus on enlightenment, with founder Nassim Haramein
- In5d: Esoteric Metaphysical and Spiritual database has resources for articles and videos about spiritual awakening, meditation, and more
- Life Purpose Help: Rev. Sandy West, life purpose coaching, reading, and healing program
- Krystal Singer: Rev. Melissa Higginbotham, practical spirituality, sound healer, singer/composer
- *Spirituality & Health* magazine: Exploring the spiritual journey—the journey to self-knowledge, authenticity, and integration, drawn from many traditions and cultures, and emphasizing sharing spiritual practices, and mind, body, and spirit exploration

The global hunger and yearning for spirituality/New Thought philosophy, mysticism, and community, and a call to action to find a deeper life purpose is permeating the educational system. Universities and institutes with educational systems specifically geared toward spiritual awakening are very popular.

Founders of Oneness University, located in India, Sri Amma and Sri Bhagavan have dedicated their lives to helping people lead fulfilled lives. The Oneness University has a large and growing international following. Oneness is a phenomenon. The purpose of the Oneness University is to spread the spirit of oneness on the planet. It starts by discovering oneness in oneself, oneness in the family, oneness in society, and oneness in the country. Then one discovers oneness on the planet and oneness toward all living things in the Universe and finally oneness with the Divine. They believe the problem of today's world is that there is no oneness within, and individual transformation leads to global transformation. So when one discovers oneness, the world discovers oneness, helping problems dissolve, which is the purpose of Oneness. Giving Oneness Deeksha has become a world phenomenon, sourced in the deep passion, intent, and spiritual sadhanas (a means of accomplishment, and ego-transcending spiritual practice) of Sri Amma and Sri Bhagavan.

Oneness Deeksha is a divine energy transfer that brings about growth in consciousness, thus heightening one's life experience. Deeksha catalyzes the secular and spiritual evolution of individuals and communities through a neurobiological shift brought about by a Divine energy transfer. It transcends religious and cultural barriers, does not bind one to any philosophy or ideology, and people belonging to any faith can receive Deeksha. Deeksha increases creative potentials; resolves inner conflict, leading to inner peace and harmony; brings love to relationships; evokes a sense of connectedness with others; heals the mind and body and evokes positive energy; and increases the abundance mentality, starts the journey into unconditional love and Awakening and God realization (onenessuniversity.org).

Emerson Theological Institute is the educational arm of Affiliated New Thought Network (ANTN), and a division of the Positive Living Center in Oakhurst, California. It is headquartered near beautiful Yosemite National

Park and is under the direction of Dr. Angelo Pizelo, its founder and director. Since its beginnings in 1992, Emerson has promoted an understanding and embodiment of the Universal Principles so that each person can pursue unlimited spiritual, emotional, intellectual, and social potential (emersoninstitute.edu).

Now, more than two decades later, Emerson and its many affiliated centers located throughout the United States and the world continue to stand for these principles embodied in its many graduates. Emerson graduates truly believe that by changing their thinking they can positively change their lives—everything is possible! Emerson Institute focuses on programs designed to further the Institute's vision of awakening people to empowering Universal Principles and providing educational resources to facilitate development of healthy relationships, spiritual communities, and realization of potential. Emerson's core curriculum embraces the spiritual ideology of the presence of God in all life and the power of right thinking, emphasizing the existence of one life, one mind, one presence in, as, and through all creation (emersoninstitute.edu).

The common emphasis of New Thought is on Universal Principles and the sacred unity of all life, oneness, and the concept that every thought manifests reality—positive and negative. Thoughts are a powerful seed to the reality that happens.

Overcoming fear and negativity, and changing your thought patterns can change your life. We must frame our thoughts in a positive frame of reference. Helping the patient frame thought patterns in the positive can be a way to assist in setting the patients' intention. When a patient makes negative statements such as, "I don't know if I will ever survive this hip fracture, I wish I would just die," teach them to rephrase to "When I recover from this hip fracture I will return home and be independent again." By making intelligent use of the subjective mind, we attract what we truly want through mind. Fear is so strong in certain health-challenging situations and patients need help to see the possible positive outcomes.

This does not mean that we have perfect lives. It means that we face the challenges of life in a way that takes the lessons and consequences of our thoughts and actions to a higher level for the next challenge. We as human beings are constantly evolving in our consciousness.

Science shows that everything in the universe is made up of energy in different shapes and forms. Energy is the building block of all matter. The same energy that makes up our bodies is the same that composes the trees, the gardens, and the waves. At one-mind-one-energy-com, Camillo Loken says, "We are all made of the same stuff. It is constantly flowing, changing form all the time, permeating everything. We are all part of one-energy". Science and spirituality are uniting in several theories in the world of physics. Basically, they hold that consciousness is required in order for particles to become reality. "Science and mysticism describe a force that connects everything together. We have the power to influence how matter behaves—and reality itself—simply through the way we perceive the world around us" (Loken, www.one-mind-one-energy.com, 2015).

All matter is energy in vibration at different frequencies. What seems to be solid matter is actually energy at a lower vibrational frequency. Humans vibrate at different levels depending on thought patterns. Our consciousness determines our level of vibration (frequency and amplitude). When we raise our thought patterns to a positive level, we increase our frequency and amplitude. Our vibration resonates out to others and attracts like vibrations. We see and understand at a higher level, a higher plane, and attract higher-level energy around us. We raise our consciousness level by vibration. The Universal Intelligence, Spirit, vibrates at the highest frequency possible, which is all-knowing, all-seeing, pure love and light.

Illness is directly associated with a perception of disconnection with the universe (only an illusion because we are all one and always connected), which makes the human energy vibration unbalanced or lower. Vibrational energy healing or harmonic healing dates back to ancient times, and a vibrational healer can influence the body and energy field by changing its frequency. "Vibrational medicine or Energy Medicine is based on the scientific principles that all matter vibrates to a precise frequency and that by using resonant vibration, balance and matter can be restored" (www.energyandvibration.com, 2015).

The goal for practitioners is to be the light that shines and vibrates truth and love with patients and clients. God speaks through many teachers, East and West, ancient and contemporary. God doesn't have a religion. God is in all religions and spiritual paths. It is not our job to teach religion to patients. It is our job as practitioners to connect deeply enough to our patients to help them connect to their own personal spirituality. I love this Hindu proverb:

There are hundreds of paths up the mountain, all leading in the same direction, so it doesn't matter which path you take. The only one wasting time is the one who runs around and around the mountain, telling everyone else that their path is wrong.

Practitioners can help patients to understand their inherent connection to the whole, as an ultimate and energetic piece of the puzzle that fits into the fabric of our cosmic community. Help patients see their value to the world and reconnect to their spirituality and we have patients who see how to become well in mind, body, and spirit.

4

Be Brave and Authentic: Therapeutic Use of Self

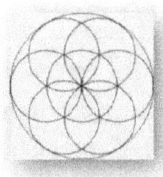

In the universe there is an immeasurable, indescribable force which shamans call intent, and absolutely everything that exists in the entire cosmos is attached to intent by a connecting link.

~CARLOS CASTANEDA

Like it or not, every single act we commit affects and influences our cosmic community, like ripples on a pond. Regardless of age, a cosmic web of unity and compassion connects us all in one big continuum. What we say and what we do, in every interaction, really does matter. We just need to remember who we are, the truth of our higher being, and bring love and light into all our interactions with one another as we each bring our unique gifts to share with the world. Bravery is being awake, staying awake, and living consciously. Awakening means coming out of the fog of rote living, paying attention, and seeing the beauty and connectivity in all things. Being authentic is to bring your whole and pure self to the table of life with soul integrity. Your whole and pure self is what is left when you peel the onion of your personality back while you remove and unlearn any negative self-images, self-doubt, and untruths you learned as a child from misguided teachers, family, and friends. Shed all fear and doubt and come alive. Bring your authentic heart-self to the path of sacred action. This is the pure you as an adult making the choice to unlearn false truths in order to be a kinder, more centered, and better human being. Walt Whitman said, "Reexamine all you have been told. Dismiss what insults your soul."

Conscious living is equivalent to knowing for sure that every single one of us is a valuable and integral part of the whole. It is living your truth and continuously clearing out negative thought patterns through constant self-reflection so you can bring your whole and higher self to the world and shine your unique light. It is discovering what you believe deep down, and erasing old hurts and insecurities you learned in childhood. Through conscious living, our positive attitude, respectful interactions, and compassion illuminate this continuum moment to moment, sending good ripples traveling afar, and making a lasting cosmic footprint of energy in the universe. Howard Thurman says, "Don't ask what the world needs. Ask what makes you come alive, and go do it. Because what the world needs is people who have come alive."

Integrity, authenticity, honesty, kindness, and our willingness to apologize easily and forgive quickly are the keys to good ripples. Find yourself and your true path, work on growth to maintain your unique self, and continuously remember who you are. Hold on to those people who nurture you and make you smile, and where possible avoid those who do not serve your best interests and higher self. Keep an open mind to the deepest parts of who you are on the inside, to your connection to the truth of your understanding as we are all constantly growing. We have the ability to empower one another through all the challenges and transitions that life brings. Bring love into all daily interaction. Focus on sending good ripples, living consciously, and leaving a lasting cosmic footprint of energy in the world that will travel forever. In sharing our stories, we help one another become all we can be on the path of sacred action.

Therapeutic Use of Self

Therapeutic use of self is defined as a practitioner's "planned use of his or her personality, insights, perceptions, judgments, as part of the therapeutic process" (Punwar and Peloquin 2000, 653). Occupational therapy practitioners cultivate and bring about rapport with patients, and build relationships through clinical knowledge, perception, empathy, compassion, and setting intentions. It is our job to bring the "big-picture thinking" to our patients. This is what we bring to the table without necessarily being conscious of it—the genuine caring, warmth, empathy, as well as the following:

- The tough love needed to wake a patient up from self-delusion
- Conveyance of our clinical expertise, and the teaching and concrete instruction needed to make it understood
- Deeper connection with the patient to elicit the trust and credibility that patients need to feel from us
- Rapport...to deep listening...to sacred connection...to sacred action
- Speaking through the spiritual common language, seeing through the spiritual lens
- Setting the intention to cultivate and allow Divine guidance in communicating rightly to each individual patient so that you draw that individual out and connect
- Keeping patients in the now

Patients bring their life experience, which includes current attitude, possible fears (Will they try to keep me here in this nursing home/hospital? Will my family forget me? Will I die here?), and family dynamics—positive and negative, pain, and possible frustration with the health-care system, workers, and doctors.

Rapport involves the *shared* experience between therapist and patient. Sometimes when a practitioner wants a patient to participate in an activity such as puzzles, crafts, or activities of daily living to elicit cognitive function, range of motion, or the ability to adapt a dressing skill, what patients sometimes really need is to be heard. How are they feeling? What is bothering them? Are they feeling disconnected? How can you empower someone if you ignore his or her worries? Shared pain eases the worries. Let them share their story.

Have you ever had the experience where the patient and you, in the noisy gym full of other patients, were so involved in a deep conversation that all distraction was like white noise magically removed from the environment, as if you were in the middle of the Mojave Desert alone together, and the gentle wind gracing your cheeks carried the beautiful desert smell of rain? This is an example of where the practitioner and patient have connected on such a deep level that time seems to stop and awareness of the now is foremost. This is deep listening. To change from treating to caring (Gawande 2014), we grow from rapport, to deep listening, to sacred connection, to sacred action. This is how we realize our greater purpose.

Nowhere is it more important for your own strong personal connection to the universe than when you are treating patients. It is your moral and ethical obligation to bring your whole self to the table. Leave your problems, complaints, and hurts, and issues with your employer, coworker, spouse, partner, or family at home. Center yourself through meditation, spiritual practices, joyful contemplation, and regular self-reflection and realignment of your sacred intention.

We need to be completely present with the human beings before us whose lives we are about to change for the better with our therapeutic knowledge base, in a loving, safe, compassionate atmosphere with humor, positivity, dignity, and deep listening. We have one common purpose: setting the intention every day to provide a culture of empowerment and tools for success so our patients can return to being as independent as possible. Our goal is to provide *sacred roots* and *wings*:

Roots in everyday living, which includes cognitive strategies, safety, balance, strength, positioning, mobility, and adaptive strategies for dressing, bathing, eating, swallowing, memory, and problem solving, including strategies to help make the reconnection to mind, body, and most important, spirit—the vital component to, and root of, absolutely knowing one's inherent connection to the whole.

Wings to go forth with a greater quality of life in connection to the Universe, focused on ability rather than disability, acceptance, and peace.

We serve with vision, positivity, and passion in order to celebrate the best in people. We choose to believe, see, and focus on the possibilities and hope that we inspire our patients to do the same. We desire to make the world a better place of unity, one patient at a time, with roots and wings.

To bring our whole self, our best therapeutic self to the table, we have reverence for all those we encounter throughout the day. We hold all paths to Truth—all wisdom, all religions, all faiths, and all agnostic and atheist belief systems—without bias. Reverence, a feeling of profound awe, respect, and honor, is a virtue that *prepares us to understand that we belong to one another.* How can anyone be hurtful to someone for whom they have reverence?

As human beings, we all have stressors that complicate our days. Patients have frustrations of not being as independent as they once were, of facing their changing circumstances, and the fear of permanently losing independence or not getting stronger fast enough. Practitioners choose to have the ultimate responsibility in meeting patients' unique needs. Remembering who we are, in our innermost higher self, and staying centered in that personal connection so we are authentic in bringing our whole self to the therapy setting, as we see each and every patient with reverence, *prepares us to belong to one another.*

Seeking and maintaining a spiritual level is finding and maintaining our level of awareness about the connections all around us such that we no longer feel separate. This requires regular self-reflection. We need to recognize with our whole being our connection to everyone and everything. The remembrance of this mystical phenomenon is that we have always been connected with the oneness of the Universe.

There are levels of awareness of wakefulness. Some people are born awake. For some, a transformational experience, catalyst, or wake-up call/event can cause a person to be awakened. The spiritual journey and awakening is different and unique for everyone. A lifelong spiritual path consisting of small steps of knowing and finding who you are can suddenly take a leap in an "aha" moment. There is no judgment about whatever level of awareness you are at. It is all about self-acceptance, self-love, and being OK with where you are. Everyone has to start somewhere. And as human beings, we all feel separate at times when we are in a funk. Having a strong connection in your path helps you get back to the connection more quickly.

Making a concerted effort to seek like-minded individuals to support your path of truth that is right for your personal belief system and keeping positive people around you help you to stay centered. Creating a sacred space for yourself or enjoying a favorite sacred place—the beach or mountains—and visiting them often, meditation and mindfulness techniques, literally smelling the flowers, enjoying music, and staying grateful in your unique connection are vital to keeping the reverence and compassion for yourself so you can have the capacity to have an authentic reverence and compassion for others.

Bring the practice from meditation into daily life: practice the awareness of breath between phone calls; practice smiling while cutting vegetables; practice relaxation after hours of hard work (Thich Nhat Hanh 1992). We need to practice self-compassion. Remember to take time to participate in whatever brings you peace. "You are here to enable the divine purpose of the universe to unfold. That is how important you are!" (Tolle 1999, preface)

Having a gratitude journal keeps the focus on being happy with what you have. Setting your intention every day to have a profound connection to your colleagues and patients and bring your best self to the therapy setting is a way to have the seed of thoughts become your reality and the reality for your patients.

5

Therapeutic Activity Integration Overview

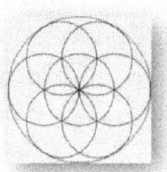

The privilege of a lifetime is being who you are.

~Joseph Campbell

Occupational therapy has long recognized the influence of the cultural and virtual context and environment on people's behavior and therefore used environmental strategies to support participation in occupation. Recognizing that for patients to truly achieve meaning and purpose, there is a unique combination of context, virtual and cultural, and environmental adjunct interventions that can promote engagement (Hooper and Wood 2014).

Successful therapeutic interventions practitioners can employ to promote spiritual connection uniquely meaningful to the individual, include, but are not limited to, gratitude, meditation, mindfulness, guided meditation, music, aromatherapy, pet therapy, gardening, creativity, and humor. Use your imagination and deep inquiry with each patient to discover his or her passion, and make that the focus to reconnection.

Simply incorporating simple spiritual interview questions within every regular screening or evaluation is an excellent best practice. Examples include asking the following: Is spirituality or religion is important to you? How well are the resources from your spiritual family working right now? Are you currently experiencing any spiritual distress? I personally like open ended questions as opposed to formal assessments as spirituality is a sensitive subject and formal assessments can be dry and impersonal. The goal of incorporating spiritual interview questions that are open ended is to generate deep rapport and sacred connection, which leads to discussion that can help assess spiritual history and help the practitioner understand and open the spiritual dialogue, ultimately empowering patients to find inner resources of healing and acceptance (Puchalski et al., 2009) through the practitioner's sacred action.

Specific examples of real-life adjunct therapeutic interventions in the form of vignettes will appear beginning in Chapter 16.

6

Therapeutic Activity Integration Overview: Gratitude

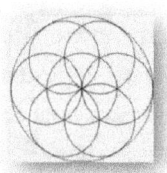

Gratitude is the memory of the heart.

~Jean Baptiste Massieu, French translation

Gratitude practice is a highly effective strategy for patient education and helping him or her connect to everyday gratitude. It is one thing to be grateful for the good things that happen to us, which most people can agree to easily. Taking gratitude to a deeper level in a therapeutic setting to foster a greater connection to the universe is a gift when patients are struggling with illness, depression, fear, pain, loss, and being estranged from a familiar setting. Practicing gratitude deeply will lead to gratitude as part of the universal flow no matter what the challenges are, and patients will feel more fullness of the heart.

Keeping a gratitude journal, writing a thank-you letter, or taking gratitude walks are three simple ways to acknowledge and practice gratitude. "Gratitude is a fullness of the heart that moves you from limitation and fear to expansion and love. When you're appreciating something, your ego moves out of the way. You can't have your attention on ego and gratitude at the same time" (Chopra, www.spiritualityhealth.com, 2015).

Integrating past and present instances of gratitude establishes a gratitude attitude and a gratitude habit. Acknowledging and integrating gratitude remembrances of the past expands the gratitude of the present and takes the focus from the current challenge we are facing to a higher connection and expectation of hope and gratitude for the future. Gratitude is globally beneficial for all people from all walks of life. In addition, this powerful remembrance practice helps in recognizing Divine grace in everyday living. Past and present gratitude begin to merge into a cosmic flow. The small things start jumping out as grace.

Even in Alzheimer's care, there are life-affirming realities. Emotional memory stays intact with even late-stage dementia. Dementia patients may not be cognitively aware of feelings or able to express them in words, but the emotion of how the caregiver makes them feel is there. They may not remember who we are, but they have a sense of how we make them feel. We can make a difference with a smile, a touch, a moment of connection. We can have gratitude that we had even a moment with a patient where we made a difference.

7

Therapeutic Activity Integration Overview: Meditation

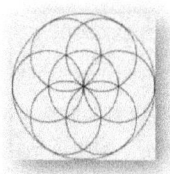

Meditation is the soul's perspective glass.

~Owen Feltham

Meditation is the personal search for meaning through engaging in deep thought or spiritual contemplation and introspection. The origin comes from 1550–1560; Latin *meditatus,* past participle of *meditari,* to meditate, contemplate, plan (Dictionary.com). "Meditation is really nondoing" (Kabat-Zinn 1990, 60). Meditation is observing the breath as we breathe in and out, giving full attention to the breath, and redirecting the attention back to the breath when the mind wanders. "A lot of meditation is about self-discovery. We start with training of attention, but attention is not the end goal of most meditation traditions; the true end goal is insight" (Tan 2012, 46).

John Kabat-Zinn and Richard Davidson conducted a study in a business setting that compared meditation groups and non-meditation groups. Measurable anxiety levels were significantly lower in the meditation group after only eight weeks of mindfulness meditation training. Electrical activity in the subject's brains was measured, and those in the meditation group showed increased activity in the area of the brain associated with positive emotions compared to the nonmeditation group. Those in the meditation group also developed more antibodies to the vaccine than the nonmeditators after flu shots were given. Meditators were measurably happier, and increased their immune system just after eight weeks of training (Tan 2012).

The types of cultural meditation traditions are vast, and a form of the practice exists in all spiritual traditions. From http://www.buddagroove.com/meditation-in-different-traditions/, below are a few examples:

- The Baha'i faith promotes meditation as the gateway for uniting oneself with the divine forces present in the universe
- In Buddhism, meditation is the core principle.
- Christian meditation centers the individual on intense prayer and contemplation to bring one closer to the Divine
- In Taoism, meditation is the key to insight and qi (natural force).
- In Hinduism, the practice of meditation is to unite with the infinite force and often involves the use of prayer beads.
- Islam/Sufism explores meditation as a pathway to awareness, creativity, and healing for divine inspiration.
- Jainism meditation inspires self-realization and salvation to become pure of heart and mind.
- Secular traditions embrace nonreligious meditation as a means for cognitive and social health.

"While symbols, tools, and mantras we place within practice may vary, the importance lies in the search itself, and our desire to connect, or perhaps reconnect, with the true self and its place in the universal system" (http://www.buddagroove.com/meditation-in-different-traditions/)

Meditation is a practice that appears in all cultures. In an effort to unite humanity, healing, and peace in all of us, there are many established efforts to unite the world in unified meditation to heal ourselves and our planet, and to uplift global consciousness. One example is at http://www.worldmeditationday.com, which promotes a world meditation day on Sundays, to meditate at any time during the twenty-four-hour period, even if only sitting and sending love and positive feelings to your surroundings. Deepak Chopra and Oprah Winfrey have a twenty-one-day meditation challenge that they offer free to the public. The founders at http://www.bethepeace.com have established a yearly meditation/prayer day since 1982, which occurs on September 21 every year at noon local time (regardless of where you live), a synchronized moment of world peace to unify the planet.

Many efforts to unite the world through synchronized meditation practice is based on the basic belief that our powerful thoughts unite us as connected beings, that as we are all one, and as one, we can change the world, one person at a time. Meditation is gaining greater respect as a modality in mainstream medicine, and the magnificence of meditation is that it can be used across the cultural, religious, and spiritual continuum as a way to bring awareness back to a patient or client's connection to Spirit, meaning, and purpose to effect healing in mind, body, and spirit.

8

Therapeutic Activity Integration Overview: Mindfulness Meditation

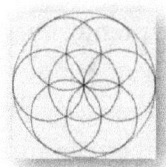

When you look at the sun during your walking meditation, the mindfulness of the body helps you to see that the sun is in you; without the sun there is no life at all and suddenly you get in touch with the sun in a different way.

~THICH NHAT HANH

Mindfulness, a form of meditation originally developed in the Buddhist traditions of Asia, is a simple and yet particularly effective tool to teach patients in a health-care setting. Mindfulness consists of focusing awareness on the present moment, while experiencing total acceptance of one's feelings and thoughts, and paying attention to all the senses. When the day gets overwhelming, one practice is to sit outside for a few minutes, feeling the cool breeze and smelling the earth, and almost tasting that beauty, hearing the trees sway and/or the creek running in the distance, and seeing the beauty around. Be one with the moment completely. This brings immediate peace among the chaos of a stressful day. "The whole essence of Zen consists in walking along the razor's edge of Now—to be so utterly, so completely *present,* that no problem, no suffering, nothing that is not *who you are* in your essence, can survive in you. In the now, in the absence of time, all your problems dissolve. Suffering needs time; it cannot survive in the Now" (Tolle 1999, 52)

The stress of managing an illness can be detrimental to the body due to the fight-or-flight response of the sympathetic nervous system. The body cannot tell the difference between a perceived threat—anxiety, the perception of spiritual disconnection, fear of health decline or death—and an actual threat, such as finding oneself next to a shark while swimming in the ocean or a seeing a bear on a hiking trail around the bend. The body suffers equally under either situation. Mindfulness has an immediate calming effect, and practiced throughout the day can relieve suffering on a permanent basis.

Mindfulness is a powerful therapeutic strategy to help patients reconnect to awareness of the Universe or the God of their understanding, bring them into the present moment where they can focus on the now instead of worry, pain, stress, or fear. "The quality of connection within us and between us and the outside worlds determine our capacity for self-regulation and healing. And the quality of those connections is maintained and can be restored by paying attention to relevant feedback" (Kabat-Zinn 1990, 228).

Self-compassion as mindfulness can be a self-soothing tool. Simple symbolic physical gestures can be taught to patients for immediate self-comfort to bring compassionate self-love and affection to oneself in the heat of the moment. One method of self-compassion is called a "self-compassion break," a power practice from Kristin Neff, from the Emerging Women website (http://www.emergingwomen.com). Finding a way to immediately respond to the self in the middle of a challenge is a very effective practice. For example, placing both hands on the heart, feeling the warmth, pressure, and the beating heart is a gesture you can teach as a coping skill of self-compassion (http://Spiritualityhealth.com). In the same manner, we can teach taking a deep breath of gratitude and exhaling the fear to bring oneself to the present and connected knowing and remembrance of self-love and compassion.

"Conscious breathing is like drinking a glass of cool water" (Thich Nhat Hanh, 2009, 3). As we breathe in, we really feel the air filling our lungs, and without controlling our breath, we feel the breath as it actually is—long or short or shallow. As we focus our attention, it will naturally become slower and deeper (Thich Nhat Hanh 2009). "By concentrating on our breathing, 'in' and 'out,' we bring body and mind back together and become whole again. Conscious breathing is an important bridge." (Thich Nhat Hanh 1992, 9)

A walking mindful meditation can be very powerful. The goal is to walk slowly and experience the five senses in complete silence while fully aware of the now. Walking meditation is walking to enjoy walking, in the spirit of the Sanskrit word *apranihita,* which means "wishlessness" or "aimlessness." Our walking is for the experience of walking, not the destination but the journey (Thich Nhat Hanh 2009, 13). This might include feeling the cool breeze on the skin and smelling a fresh scent of the rain-soaked trees following a rainstorm, and seeing the beauty of the environment—the blue sky, greenery, the warmth of the sun, tasting the apple freshly picked from the tree, hearing the rushing creek in the distance, and touching and smelling the pine needles or leaves of the environment. This is a guided walk you can take with your patients to help them experience the oneness of nature.

I had the honor and privilege of participating in a walking meditation at Deer Park Monastery several years ago in Escondido, California, with Thich Nhat Hanh. Although there were hundreds of people on that walk, I happened to fall in right behind Thich Nhat Hanh at the beginning of the walk, and what a wonderful experience it was to watch and emulate his mindful touch on the surrounding greenery, observe how he smelled the leaves and took in the environment. It was so exciting to be part of that large group, each of us matching this master's steps and gestures to seek his teaching. His teaching of the mindful walk and being one with the moment and environment will forever be with me, an experience I will always cherish.

9

Therapeutic Activity Integration Overview: Guided Meditation

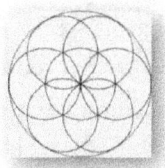

There are techniques of Buddhism, such as meditation, that anyone can adopt. And, of course, there are Christian monks and nuns who already use Buddhist methods in order to develop their devotion, compassion, and ability to forgive.

~Dalai Lama

A wonderful way to help a patient or client experience a heightened state of consciousness is to have the person close his or her eyes and experience a form of meditation called guided meditation, where we verbally guide the patient through either a live face-to-face visualization or a prerecording of a guided meditation. Guided meditation is one of the most highly effective and least complicated ways to bring a patient to a peaceful place and introduce visualization and imagination in effecting positive change. Guided meditation utilizes mental imagery or creative visualization to walk a client through a set of images of a safe place.

The patient or client is first given verbal instructions that teach him or her how to relax the body, clear the mind, concentrate on breathing, and focus awareness and attention. I have found that asking questions and using an example of a favorite sacred place is a wonderful opportunity to create a custom guided meditation designed in a similar setting. There are many resources out there for commercial prerecorded guided meditations. I prefer a custom one that aims at the individual's idea of a sacred space. For example, I had a patient who grew up in the high desert of California, so I created a guided meditation that included the high desert imagery and visualization that the patient responded to very well. Scenes from the ocean setting as a sacred space are also fun to use, because many people love the ocean.

The advantage of guided meditations as an introduction to meditation and the imaginative aspect is that it is easy for the patient or client. Guided meditation introduces the concepts that require the imagination to go to another place to relax, reduce stress, and increase spiritual awareness. Traditional meditation takes effort to stay focused and keep the mind clear. With guided meditation, the mind is guided by the word of another, who takes the client to a special place and introduces concepts that may be new and easier to grasp through the specific tour toward deep meditation. Utilizing the power of the patient or client's imagination and visualization can be even more powerful than traditional meditation, and the experience of deep inner stillness can be profound.

I recently experienced a guided meditation that took me to a place where my imagination had me sitting with and talking to God, in pure energy nonform, and feeling a complete surrender and absolute love in a way I had never experienced before. It was, and still is, a very exceptional and powerful remembrance of absolute love, Christ consciousness, and complete acceptance that I return to often in my meditation practice. Every time I remember, I feel as though it was a real experience and I experience the feeling again and again of being in the presence of and connected to Absolute Love.

10

Therapeutic Activity Integration Overview: Music Therapy

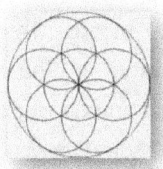

One good thing about music, when it hits you, you feel no pain.

~Bob Marley

Music is the seat of the soul. Music can help us transcend our daily lives. Music and sound are natural healing agents and have been universally used across all time and all cultures. Sound healing is based on the principle that sounds change consciousness. Sound and music can be utilized as therapeutic and transformational modalities.

If all life is consciousness, then inanimate objects such as musical instruments are a part of that consciousness on some level. "In many creation stories, you hear that in the beginning was sound, and when it moved and projected out into manifestation, it became light. Light subsequently slowed down its rotation of particle spin and became matter. So light and sound became matter, but rhythm determines the shape it takes" (Higginbotham 2014, 35)

"Music is one of the oldest forms of preventive medicine known to humanity" (Stevens 2012, 9). It can shape our personalities and behaviors, return us to vivid long-ago memories, and to the primal heartbeat rhythm from the womb. Researchers at Boston Children's Hospital found that early musical training helps improve executive functions, and "sets children up for a better academic future" (www.sciencedaily.com)

"Sound breaks up patterns of energy and allows the body the opportunity to manifest its original soul blueprint." (Higginbotham 2014, 29) Sound penetrates the life-denying patterns of energy. Sound then becomes the catalyst for penetrating and dissolving the armor of that life-denying pattern of energy for healing the mind, body, and spirit. As the outmoded patterns are lifted out, the resulting space is infused with Source energy (Higginbotham 2014).

Using music as a healing modality, the healing facilitator must start from an inner focus of wholeness, no matter what type of musical instrument is utilized, whether it is drums, crystal or Tibetan bowls, or the voice. The original Divine blueprint will be what travels out on the sound for Divine healing. "Sound is consciousness, and consciousness travels on sound" (Higginbotham 2014, 33)

Clapping and rhythm therapy are used with patients with diagnoses of cerebral vascular accident (CVA) and dementia by OTs and speech therapists (STs) alike. Like a metronome, the constant beat can help patients in many ways to keep a pace in any activity. Music can provide benefits to long-term memory. Music is used for enhancing running, ambience for sex, relaxation for yoga, creating art, and creative writing. Music is common in palliative care and has a calming and peaceful effect.

Music therapy is an activity that promotes connection to Spirit, to remember who we really are as creative vessels. Around the world, drumming and rhythm have been used in many indigenous cultures to heal. The patient is placed in the center of a circle of drummers or dancers who use their feet to provide rhythm. While focusing on wholeness, they drum and use rhythm to have a cleansing effect on the patient through the energy fields. "All life has its own inherent rhythm. In a sense you could say that illness results when your inner rhythm is off track. We use percussive instruments to bring back and re-pattern your own life rhythm" (Higginbotham 2014, 38)

Not only creating music but also playing and listening to music can be a profoundly powerful therapeutic intervention. Providing meaningful therapeutic music choices for each patient requires the OT practitioner to listen deeply to the patient or the patient's family. Understanding musical preferences is vital in the therapeutic relationship for effective therapeutic outcomes in music therapy. Simple inquiry can include the following: Do you play an instrument? What is your favorite kind of music? Did you listen to music as a child? What was a favorite music choice in your childhood home?

After discovering the patient's preferences, therapists can start with simply playing uplifting music, sacred gospel music, era music that a patient can relate to, that culminates in singing remembered songs. Another activity is a rhythm group with drums, maracas, a tambourine, handheld bells, castanets, a tone block, rhythm sticks, and so forth. "Medicine men and women used drumming and chanting to treat illnesses. Shamans were doctors in indigenous tribes, traveling on drumbeats to other realms to care for the soul's spiritual health. This connection of music and medicine continues today" (Stevens 2012, 9)

The mystery of music is why one genre brings us to our roots and another one does not. "Rhythm is the instrument of art and music is the organization, not only of rhythm but of scale and of the notes played against each other" (Osbon 1991, 249).

I have witnessed a guitar and drumming group improvise and magically come together in cadence, chords, and notes. I felt I was witness to the mystery, the creative supreme connection experience that takes on a beautiful life of its own in total abandon. What resonates for each patient is what we need to discover. As Friedrich Nietzsche said, "Without music, life would be a mistake."

Music therapy is a valuable intervention due to its ability to "offer an experience of time that is qualitatively rich" (Aldridge 1995, 107). Music can be soothing, inspiring, and uplifting. Different dimensions of music include inducing motions on the body, satisfying the intellect, adding a tendency toward beauty and grace, piercing the heart, and even inspiring the soul to the harmony of the spheres. Music helps patients find meaning and purpose, hope and faith, and quality of life (Aldridge 1995). There is healing power through music, "a process of bringing back into life what is missing; it is a process of becoming whole" (Stevens 2012, 11).

To this day, hearing music of my childhood that included folk music from the Brothers Four, Chet Atkins, and Tchaikovsky's "1812 Overture" instantly bring tears of nostalgic emotions, in fond remembrance and association to my family life in the 1960s. This was a very happy time of life for me. Music brings rich memories back to the memory surface that are associated with time and place. When I hear that music, I vividly remember the house we lived in at the time, the rich smells of the Mojave Desert, my older brothers' and my parents' laughter, and making homemade ice cream in our park-like backyard. That music has a forever connection in my psyche to my life in the 1960s. Music memory is powerful and beautiful. The music of the Brothers Four, Chet Atkins, and Tchaikovsky has the effect of bringing me to my roots, and time and place associations with my childhood and family.

Ambient music, nature-sound therapy, can "help meet social and emotional needs and reduce the problem behavior displayed by people with dementia. Active music intervention can also increase attention and orientation. The desired outcome is the modulation of agitation" (Padilla 2011, 517).

There is a world movement in skilled nursing facility (SNF) and other dementia-care settings based on the 2014 documentary *Alive Inside: A Story of Music and Memory*. Director Michael Rossato-Bennett filmed social worker Dan Cohen, MSW, for three years while he was working with patients with dementia, revealing a remarkable music-based breakthrough that has already transformed lives. Music is a key to unlocking memory. Musical memory is profoundly linked to emotions stored deep in the brain. Per the Music and Memory certification website (musicandmemory.com), "While Alzheimer's damages the ability to recall facts and details, it does not destroy the lasting connections between a favorite song and memory of an important life event, no matter how long ago." When hearing a tune connected to a meaningful memory, a person with Alzheimer's can suddenly awaken, sing lyrics, and sometimes speak when he or she has not spoken in years. With this program, a personalized playlist is created on an iPod with the specific music that the patient likes. Creating personalized playlists is a very advantageous approach when compared to having a general music group in which the music chosen may not be to the liking of everyone in the group (www.musicandmemory.com).

11

Therapeutic Activity Integration Overview: Aromatherapy

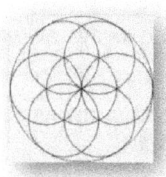

Intuition is really a sudden immersion of the soul into the universal current of life.

-PAULO COELHO, *THE ALCHEMIST*

Aromatherapy is a form of alternative medicine that uses plant materials and aromatic plant oils, including essential oils and other aromatic compounds, for the purpose of mood alteration and well-being. Per the University of Maryland Medical System Aromatherapy website (http://umm.edu/health/medical/altmed/treatment/aromatherapy), "Essential oils are concentrated extracts taken from the roots, leaves, seeds or blossoms of plants and have been used for therapeutic purposes for nearly 6000 years. The ancient Chinese, Indians, Egyptians, Greeks and Romans used them in cosmetics, perfumes, and drugs. Essential oils were also commonly used for spiritual, therapeutic, hygienic and ritualistic purposes."

Modes of application include aerial diffusion, direct inhalation, and topical applications. I prefer aerial diffusion in the occupational therapy setting. Applying essential oils topically may lead to allergic reactions, which are hard to anticipate; however, any application process is acceptable. Merely adding a drop of essential oil recipe mix to a cotton ball can be sufficient. You can find essential oils and nice diffusers at http://www.mydoterra.com/mygarden.

Aromatherapy can be a fabulous adjunct to occupational therapy. It may reduce anxiety, enhance memory, increase relaxation, decrease pain, and alleviate headaches and insomnia, among many other benefits. As a whole, studies suggest that aromatherapy may be useful in inducing relaxation, and reducing agitation and sleep fragmentation, all common in people with dementia. Aromatherapy has also been effective in reducing sundowning syndrome, a late-day and evening state of confusion that sometimes brings behaviors such as agitation, anxiety, aggression, and wandering in residents with dementia, and nocturnal agitation. Aromatherapy is one of the most widely applied complementary therapies used for people with dementia.

Another pilot study using essential oils in the classroom with children with autism and autism spectrum disorders found that "essential oils can instantly affect the behavior of the autistic child in the classroom setting. The most successful oils in calming and focusing were cinnamon bark and benzoin. The children fidgeted less, were more likely to listen, and were more involved in question-and-answer games with benzoin, frankincense, and cinnamon. Bergamot and neroli had a calming effect; however, the children continued to fidget. Bergamot and cinnamon elicited more smiles, jokes, and generally a happier atmosphere" (Meulman, www.healingmuse.com, 2009).

Aromatherapy is an especially important adjunct therapy approach in patients with dementia who exhibit behavioral or psychotic symptoms common to dementia such as anxiety, aggression (verbal and/or physical), confusion, and the sometimes out-of-control behavior that is not only distressing to the patient but also to the caregivers. The first line of treatment is commonly pharmacological, with neuroleptic agents. "Neuroleptics can be poorly tolerated by people with dementia, particularly among those with severe dementia, and there is a high risk of adverse events (e.g., Parkinsonism, drowsiness, falls, accelerated cognitive decline, increased mortality), and a detrimental impact upon key indicators of quality of life, including activities, well-being, and social interaction" (Ballard, O'Brien, Reichelt, and Perry 2002, 4).

In a double-blind, placebo-controlled trial at Wolfson Research Centre Institute for Ageing and Health in Newcastle upon Tyne, United Kingdom, 60 percent of the treatment group patients with severe dementia experienced overall improvement in levels of agitation and significant improvement in quality of life with Melissa lemon balm essential oil. The conclusion of the study was that aromatherapy with essential balm is safe (Ballard et al. 2002).

You can buy eyedroppers, vegetable carrier oil (I like the sweet almond), and small blue bottles for the purpose of mixing your own, which can be more economical. Examples of carrier oils include almond, hazelnut, grape-seed, soy, peanut, peach apricot kernel, avocado, and wheat germ. You can Google "essential oils" to find many suppliers in your area who sell essential oils and supporting equipment, if you choose to mix your own. You can also order premixed recipes of essential oils and basic essential oils from places such as http://www.mydoterra.com/mygarden and http://www.lotionlady.com. Aromatherapy is also going mainstream in many skilled nursing facility chains, large and small, and other dementia settings.

A few examples of aromatherapy recipes that I have used as adjunct therapy in the SNF setting with success are listed in the table below.

Concentration and Memory	10 drops grapefruit, 8 drops basil, 7 drops lavender, 5 drops rosemary, 2 Tbsp. sweet almond carrier oil
Insomnia	10 drops clary sage, 10 drops sandalwood, 10 drops lemon, 2 Tbsp. sweet almond carrier oil
Anxiety	15 drops geranium, 5 drops lavender, 10 drops bergamot, 2 Tbsp. sweet almond carrier oil
Headaches	3 drops lavender, 1 drop peppermint, 1 Tbsp. sweet almond carrier oil
Muscle Stiffness	10 drops marjoram, 10 drops rosemary, 5 drops basil, 5 drops lemon, 2 Tbsp. sweet almond carrier oil

12

Therapeutic Activity Integration Overview: Pet Therapy

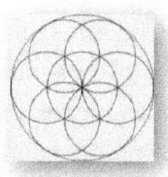

Humanity is exalted not because we are so far above other living creatures, but because knowing them well elevates the very concept of life.

~Edward O. Wilson

Pet therapy is a general term that includes a growing field that uses dogs or other animals to help people cope and recover from health problems, including heart issues, mental health issues, and cancer diagnoses. In addition, the term includes animal-assisted activities, which provide comfort and enjoyment for hospital patients and nursing home residents (Mayo Clinic 2015). "Research has shown pet ownership reduces blood pressure, and other risk factors for heart disease and improves social and psychological functioning" (Zisselman, Rovner, Shmuely and Ferrie 1996, 47).

Pets provide unconditional, nonjudgmental love, companionship, attention, forgiveness, and affection. Animals can shift our narrow focus beyond ourselves, helping us to feel connected to the Universe and create a sense of being needed for the geriatric population. Further benefits of animal-assisted therapy include increased sensory stimulation through petting, improved sense of purpose, companionship, improved self-esteem, and increased social interaction among staff and residents (Fick 1993).

Because the geriatric population often withdraws from social interaction and sometimes self-isolate due to decreased mobility or other health issues and relies more on the virtual environment, they have great potential in benefitting from animal-assisted therapy. Animal-assisted therapy also helps with reality orientation, decreasing isolation, increased socialization, communication, anxiety levels, attention span, and engagement (Fick 1993).

When people are in a nursing home, assisted living or hospital setting, animal-assisted therapy can provide the comfort that reminds them of current or past pets. Pets can reduce stress-induced symptoms such as anxiety and fear, and can add years to one's life, regardless of the type of pet. Animal-assisted therapy can significantly reduce pain, anxiety, depression, and fatigue in people with various health problems, including, but not limited to, people in cancer treatment, in long-term care facilities, with heart failure, and veterans with posttraumatic stress disorder (PTSD). In addition, their family members benefit as well when the animals visit. Pet therapy is also being used in nonmedical settings such as community programs that help people deal with stress and anxiety (Mayo Clinic 2015).

Animals must be vaccinated, trained, and screened for appropriate behavior or infection. Hospitals, rehabilitation units, and SNFs have stringent rules for pets, so make sure you follow the rules of your particular unit. There are many community programs that reach out to health-care settings such as SNF, assisted living, hospital, and dementia units to provide this type of therapy. You can research your community to find one you can partner with—one that will make regular visits.

13

Therapeutic Activity Integration Overview: Gardening

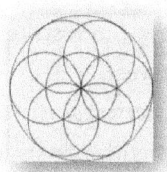

*I once had a sparrow alight upon my shoulder for a moment,
while I was hoeing in a village garden, and I felt that I was
more distinguished by that circumstance than I should have
been by any epaulet I could have worn.*

~Henry David Thoreau

Gardening can bring back rich memories of childhood, and digging in the dirt often becomes a spiritual experience, breeding optimism and hope. Gardening can bring peace and solitude—a perfect place for mindfulness as one feels the soil, the scent of earth, and the water. Camaraderie and bonding often develop among a garden group. The garden area can become a place of refuge, a sacred space to go to relax, read a book, watch insects, be one with nature, and increase happiness (Park and VanLeit 2012).

Gardening is a life-nurturing undertaking that reaffirms spiritual source and spiritual cultivation as the act of gardening occurs. Gardening is an ongoing cycle that affirms hope and grace in the bounty of the seasons, each season a part of the spiritual process. In gardening we trust the universe. The seed knows what to do. We become one with the garden as we co-create *with* it and witness the seasons that parallel the circle of life that we share. It becomes a partnership of life and rebirth. Providing a garden to work in at any physical or mental disability level is a life-affirming and powerful therapeutic intervention for well-being in general, and for healing and a sense of connection to Spirit.

Accessible raised garden beds are perfect for wheelchair access in nursing home and assisted living settings or even at home. Gardening gets residents/patients outdoors, under the sun, and into the fresh air, thus promoting better sleep. An ongoing gardening group can have the full experience of planting, tilling, watching the garden grow, harvesting the vegetables, and then finally, a cooking group to serve the harvest.

In addition, I suggest partnering with the community garden club for lectures and visual presentations and scheduling field trips to local gardens for residents to enjoy the beauty and fresh air in a professional garden atmosphere.

Finally, post gardening activity discussions regarding the benefits or the memories that the activity brought gives an opportunity to reinforce the spiritual aspect of the experience and the mindfulness techniques that can be practiced in the next outdoor session.

14

Therapeutic Activity Integration Overview: Creativity

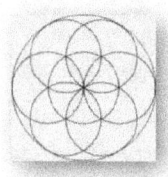

When I open my eyes in the morning, I am not confronted by the world, but by a million possible worlds.

~COLIN WILSON

Creativity is a direct connection to Spirit. "Creativity is a powerful shaping force in human life. It is an intangible human capacity of a transcendent nature—it moves us beyond ourselves in a similar way to spirituality" (Paintner 2007, 2). A painting, dance, or story that previously had not existed before is the result of bringing new and imaginative ideas into reality. The root of creativity is in the soul. The Divine connection is where inspiration is derived. Author and anthropologist Ellen Dissanayake even suggests that "the act of creating is actually biological need that is basic to human nature." (Paintner, 2007, 2)

"Carl Jung believed images are expressions of deep human experience and our authentic selves. They are the natural and primary language for the psyche, and only secondarily do we move to conceptual thought. Jung saw images as clues to the unlived life that move toward some form of outward expression and urged others to look at the images of their lives in a symbolic way so as to reveal deeper meanings and their fuller, more authentic selves" (Paintner, 2007, 2)

The imagination is essential to humanness, involving creative, intuitive, and integrative processes relating to becoming. "It gives us the power to remember the past, to shape our desires, and to project the possibilities for the future" (Paintner, 2007, 3) Creativity is at the heart of being human, to be able to determine our future, have satisfying relationships, play, form new opportunities in the workplace, and create new dreams for ourselves, families, communities, our world, and the universe (Paintner, 2007).

During the creative process, the body releases natural opiates, making the creative process intrinsically rewarding. "You get these little shots of dopamine in the reward centers of the brain," says Shelley Carson, author of *Your Creative Brain: Seven Steps to Maximize Imagination, Productivity, and Innovation in Your Life* (Haupt 2015, 3) Dopamine is a mood-elevating neurotransmitter that is released with pleasurable experiences such as food, sex, and drugs—and creativity (Haupt 2015, 3).

The inner self is the spiritual self, where creativity spins directly from source—the Absolute. Using a holistic approach to therapy, promoting creativity can help a patient or client to explore his or her motivations and feelings, and help increase and develop empowerment. Creativity also can bring back the wonderment in life. It helps us adapt to new realities and bridge the perceived lost connections. Painting, drawing, making collages, dancing, and writing in journals are some strategies for promoting creativity and a sense of reconnection. Therapeutic interventions like these can be in groups and individual treatment.

The healing power of creative therapy is a potent therapeutic tool. "Art therapy shifts the focus to creating, enjoying, and sharing positive stimuli" (Haupt 2015, 3). Patients and clients enjoy chosen colors and textures, and sharing feelings and finished projects in a group. The joyful experience from creating and sharing as a spiritual practice is a Divine intervention.

There are many ways to empower patients, residents, or clients in creativity. It does not have to be expensive. Simple collages based on a theme, with donated magazines, can be powerful, yet inexpensive, tools for creativity activities. For example, in using images of empowerment as a theme, I worked with a resident who was in a battered women's shelter, and she made a collage of female characters that embodied power—Wonder Woman, an Annie Oakley look-alike picture, and Joan of Arc. It was very empowering for her. For fine art, you can utilize colored pencils and watercolors. Local artist communities may be willing to donate supplies.

Dancing can be a simple line dance, which is a fun way to get clients in tune with their bodies without the pressure of performance anxiety. Free-form jazz dancing can also be fun in certain settings.

Simple composition books from the dollar store work well for creative writing or journal writing. The focus is not on quality but the process and valuable connections to feelings, empowerment, and a sense of remembering who the clients are as spiritual human beings. Think outside the box as you get to know your patient, resident, or client. There are many ways to be creative.

15

Therapeutic Activity Integration Overview: Humor

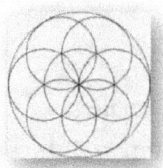

The kind of humor I like is the thing that makes me laugh for five seconds and think for ten minutes.

~WILLIAM DAVIS

It is often said that laughter is the best medicine. Laughing at the good things and learning to laugh at the bad things can be therapeutic. "Spirituality is in all things, and that includes humor. Life is a funny, wild, and ridiculous adventure as much as it is serious, deep, or tragic at times. So we all learn the importance of laughing and enjoying the silliness that we create and that is presented to us. With humor, we are enacting happiness" (Tolles, www.spiritualawakeningprocess.com 2012).

"The purpose of our existence is to seek happiness" (Dalai Lama and Cutler, 1998, 16). Seeking Happiness is not self-centered by nature. Surveys show that "it is *unhappy* people who tend to be most self-focused and are often socially withdrawn, brooding, and even antagonistic. Happy people, in contrast, are more sociable, flexible, and creative and are able to tolerate life's daily frustrations more easily than unhappy people." (Dalai Lama and Cutler 1998, 17)

They are also more loving and forgiving than unhappy people (Dalai Lama and Cutler 1998, 17).

Researchers have demonstrated that "happy people exhibit a certain quality of openness, a willingness to reach out and help others" (Dalai Lama and Cutler 1998, 17). In one scenario, a subject listened to a comedy album and experienced an uplift in spirit. Someone in need (part of the experiment), approached the subject and asked for money. The subjects who were feeling happy were more likely to help than the control group who did not get a boost ahead of time (Dalai Lama and Cutler, 1998).

Humor Is Happiness Embodied

So, what is humor, anyway? Humor is the propensity of a particular mental experience to bring about laughter and delight. There are many techniques of humor—slapstick, exaggeration, absurdity, and imitation, to name a few. Humor can also be verbal, audible, visual, and physical (King 2014).

"Jokes are actions with humorous intent" (King, 2014, 3) and take on different forms. For example, a single thought or gesture, such as the simple question, "Seriously?" or a question and answer such as "Why did the chicken cross the road?" Another example is a short story: "A guy walks into a bar…" Jokes typically reflect irony, sarcasm, or wordplay and most have a punch line (King 2014, 3).

Humor and laughter cross all cultures. Humor is important in health and wellness as a means to reduce stress and bring forth laughter. Humor can also be a defense mechanism, an "overt expression of ideas and feelings too unpleasant or terrible to talk about that gives pleasure to others" (King 2014, 4). "Laughter is both an expression of happiness and contributor to happiness." (King 2014, 4) Laughter lowers blood pressure, reduces stress hormones such as cortisol and adrenaline, helps defend against illness, and can improve memory, creativity, and learning (King 2014). Humor also activates the dopamine reward centers. Laughter is social. It strengthens relationships, promotes group bonding, facilitates cooperation and teamwork, defuses conflict, elevates the pain threshold "by breaking the cycle between pain, sleep loss, depression, and immune suppression," (King 2014, 13) and can increase one's life expectancy (King 2014).

Bringing more humor in life is more than thinking positive. Humor gives us a chance to feel it in the heart, body, and mind—a way to embody Spirit and the joy of living. We need to be able to laugh at ourselves and lighten up. For example, creating a laughing group can be a fun way to promote a spiritual practice of humor and bring patients together. Laughter is infectious. And laughter and humor can set us free. Freedom from the seriousness helps us grow spiritually. It can be as simple as having your residents/patients watch a funny movie or stand-up comedy. "Laughter and humor is a tool like meditation, journaling, and everything else. Look at the things you worry about and laugh" (Tolles, www.spiritualawakeningprocess.com, 2012).

In the 1960s, Norman Cousins used humor to heal when he contracted a rare and painful joint disease that was supposed to be a terminal illness. He did not give in to pain. Instead, he watched the Marx brothers and *Candid Camera* on television and realized that ten minutes of healing laughter would win him two hours of pain relief. He made an amazing recovery over a few months (www.solitaries.org).

16

Vignettes–Real-Life Examples: Gratitude

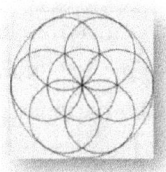

As we express our gratitude, we must never forget that the highest appreciation is not to utter words, but to live by them.

~JOHN F. KENNEDY

Gratitude work is one of the simplest activities to help patients, residents, or clients focus on their gratitude for the good in their life instead of focusing on the challenges. Remember that what is focused on in our thoughts is what the Universe hears and responds to. You cannot be focused on gratitude and be worried at the same time. A gratitude focus can bring amazing change to one's perception of reality.

- Eighty-two-year-old, right-hand-dominant female patient R.B. admitted to a SNF; status: post-cerebral vascular accident (CVA) with right hemiplegia (loss of motor function). The patient was raised Catholic and was still active in the church. The patient had strong family support with two daughters who frequently visited. On day seven of her Medicare SNF stay, the patient expressed feelings of helplessness and hopelessness, signs of depression, to her (OT). R.B. didn't want to burden her family with her feelings. The OT engaged the patient in group therapy activities with other patients of similar diagnosis. The patient continued to express signs and symptoms of depression. One day the OT asked the patient what she was most thankful for in her life. The patient had a hard time coming up with anything in the moment. The OT got out a piece of paper, and the patient agreed to come up with a list of things she was grateful for together. Every night the patient was given an assignment to think of one more item for the list, and she and the therapist would add to her list the next day. After several days the list was longer, and the patient's attitude became more positive. This list graduated to become her gratitude journal. After eliciting the patient's permission to share her feelings of hopelessness with her daughter in an occupational therapy session, the daughter who was attending the session was very positive and supportive. With family support the patient's focus stayed on the positive. The OT asked the family to call the church to which the patient belonged, and subsequently one of the nuns whom she was very fond of visited her. In group settings with other patients, R.B. began counseling other patients to stay positive and focus on the gratitude. She shared her gratitude journal with the group and challenged them to create a gratitude journal for themselves. With the help of the OT, the family, and the sister from the Catholic Church, the patient was able to redirect her focus to what she was grateful for. In addition, the daughter wrote a little song for the patient to sing every day with the lyrics focusing on gratitude:

I'm alive, awake, alert,
Relaxed, enthusiastic!
I'm alive, awake, alert,
Relaxed, enthusiastic!
And I appreciate
That I feel fantastic!
And I appreciate you and you and you!

R.B. sang this little song every time she came into the gym for ther-apy, and when she got to the last line, she pointed to each person in the gym with each "you."

Other patients followed suit with the gratitude journal, which helped them on their road to recovery. This event helped the OT to acknowledge the benefits of having a gratitude journal. The OT cre-ated a gratitude group where the patients could share their journals and help one another focus on the positive. There were very positive outcomes for increased positive attitudes, and even the staff became uplifted.

17

Vignettes–Real-Life Examples: Meditation

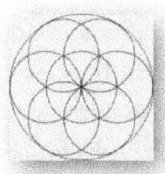

To understand the immeasurable, the mind must be extraordinarily quiet, still.

—Jiddu Krishnamurti

Meditation is much less complicated than what people think. It is such a simple tool to teach and helps patients reduce stress and anxiety, and offers great benefits to physical and mental well-being. Meditation is instrumental in facilitating and maintaining meaningful connection to Spirit based on the individual's understanding of that connection, and to those who do not believe in a higher power, maintaining a meaningful life, personal moral code, standards, and purpose.

- T.C., a sixty-six-year-old male and homeless veteran was admitted to a SNF; status: post-three-day hospitalization at the Veterans Administration (VA) hospital after being found on the street unconscious due to a diabetic episode, hypertension, nonhealing foot wound, a diagnosis of posttraumatic stress disorder (PTSD), and a history of alcohol abuse. The patient was noted to have significant weakness due to the recent hospitalization on the occupational therapy and physical therapy evaluations. The patient has a daughter and a brother whom he has not seen "in a long time," and his ex-wife was completely out of the picture due to his admitted alcohol-related behaviors. The patient presented with covert anger, inappropriate outbursts, and was resistive to therapy. Therapists from both disciplines were having issues with this veteran accepting and participating in physical therapy and occupational therapy activities.

T.C. was very upset about being confined to a wheelchair due to his non-weight-bearing status secondary to nonhealing wounds on his ankle and foot. Therapy staff asked the OT/director of rehabilitation to intervene to "get him to participate."

T.C. had matted hair and a foul odor from being on the street and was refusing to allow a shower the certified nursing assistants were offering him. The OT established a good rapport through deep listening techniques and much patience, and the patient began to trust the therapist. The OT began introducing concepts about practicing self-compassion and understanding his inherent value in the world. Over the next few treatment sessions, the veteran began to open up and was able to verbalize frustrations about his perception of "the system," and being on a waiting list for intervention with his PTSD and diabetes. He also expressed verbalizations and body language reflecting anger, anxiety, and hopelessness, and stated that "There is no God because of the horrible suffering in the world of constant wars."

After a week of the OT utilizing her deep listening skills and conveying unconditional compassion in her discussions with T.C., he began opening up about his anger and his alcohol habits. His anger had been negatively affecting his blood pressure as well. The patient's trust in the therapist continued to deepen. T.C. agreed to a shower with the assistance of the OT, and the OT was allowed to assist in shaving him; he let "only her" comb and trim his hair. He expressed "feeling like a new man" after that. Because of the OT's ability to connect with the patient, the facility called on her to intervene when the patient refused medication or other vital nursing interventions.

The OT began talking to T.C. about ways to relieve stress and deal with anxiety, which he identified as reasons for using alcohol. Meditation was introduced in its simplest form. The patient was encouraged to spend just five minutes per day in a quiet space and to allow his thoughts to flow past, without judgment, and to become an observer of the thoughts, as he focused on his breath. He was instructed to refocus on his breath every time he lost his concentration on letting the thoughts flow by.

The patient responded well to this intervention and was instructed to increase the length of time to ten minutes. On pleasant weather days, the patient began to voluntarily wheel himself outside to enjoy the sun and meditate. He increased to twenty minutes twice per day. After two more weeks, his blood pressure was under control, and he was consistently agreeing to his medication regimen with nursing staff.

He became calmer and started earnestly participating in all therapy. The OT called the local Alcoholics Anonymous chapter, and with T.C.'s permission, they sent over a veteran to work with him. With T.C.'s uplifted attitude and increasing positive therapy outcomes, he began to recover. He was able to get into a veteran's housing program upon discharge from the facility. He conveyed that meditation was the beginning of his life change, and he discharged with a positive outlook and had reconnected to his spiritual roots.

18

Vignettes–Real-Life Examples: Mindfulness

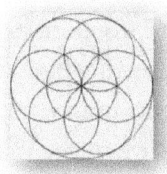

*The most precious gift we can offer anyone is our attention.
When mindfulness embraces those we love, they will bloom like
flowers.*

-Thich Nhat Hanh

Mindfulness is a wonderful tool to coach in order to guide patients to the present moment and focus on the now and appreciate what is. Mindfulness is the single most valuable means to redirect focus, by using all the senses, to the present moment. Mindfulness can be presented in individual therapy, and it also works well in groups. Being your own spontaneous presenter of the real-life environment as a guide to introduce this technique is fun!

- M.C., a seventy-two-year-old female admitted to a SNF; status: post–right total hip replacement (THR). M.C. also has a diagnosis of hypertension and diabetes, and while at the SNF developed a blistery rash on her left side that was diagnosed as shingles, a very painful nerve condition related to the chicken pox virus. M.C. enjoyed being an active senior who normally walks a few miles per day with the "neighborhood girls." She was handling the THR gallantly until she developed shingles. She was in a lot of pain.

M.C. told the OT she was very discouraged with the new onset of additional pain from the shingles and began to refuse all therapy. It was vital to continue walking in order to heal from the surgery to avoid stiffness and to keep increasing the range of motion in her new hip. The OT was able to convince her to go outside and enjoy the sun for a few minutes with her, and introduced the mindfulness concept to M.C. after she commented on how good the sun felt.

The OT asked M.C. to close her eyes, and called M.C.'s attention to the gentle breeze flowing across her face, and the warmth of the sun. M.C. was encouraged to breathe deeply and be with the sun and the breeze. A lemon tree was close by, and the lemons were rounding and ripening in bright yellow, and the waft of lemon scent was floating on top of the gentle breeze. The OT asked, "Can you smell the lemons?" M.C. nodded her head in the affirmative. "Now open your eyes and look at those tiny white buds and blooming petals on the lemon tree. Feel the deep beauty in the tree. The deep-green elongated leaves. Look at the beautiful rounding lemons. Reach out and touch the leaves. Feel the coolness of the thin leaf, the softness of the petals, and the coarse outer peel of the newly formed lemons. Experience the textures."

The OT went on. "Continue to deep breathe with your eyes open, and be with the tree, the breeze, the warmth of the sun, the lemon scent, the softness of the white petals, the coolness of the deep-green leaf, and the coarse outer lemon rounding. Just be here with all your senses, in tune to the now. Keep breathing."

The OT was able to continue this deep breathing and "now" exercise with M.C. for about twenty minutes. M.C. was in awe of the aftereffects of the exercise upon conclusion. "I didn't feel pain!" M.C. exclaimed.

M.C. liked it so much that she began coming outside and doing her own mindfulness exercises every day. This helped ease her pain, and she was willing to come back to therapy in full participation and was able to go home two weeks later with a very positive attitude.

The OT also started a mindfulness group where she went through the same steps with the group, experiencing the five senses in the now. This became a regular and popular Friday group.

- T.S. was a seventy-seven-year-old male admitted to the SNF after a myocardial infarction (MI). T.S. was discouraged at his inability to walk very far without becoming very short of breath. He never thought he would be in this position. "A heart attack! Me? This is not happening." T.S. was able to walk about a hundred feet very slowly without resting. The OT introduced him to mindfulness walking. Mindfulness walking is a way to walk very slowly in full awareness of all the senses, and to take notice of all the beauty and smells and textures along the way. This means walking leisurely and touching the vegetation, feeling the leaves, smelling and touching the flowers, enjoying the warmth of the sun and gentle breeze, and smelling the earth. She walked with him and coached him to enjoy the beauty and smells, and to reach out and experience the texture of the leaves and flowers between his fingers while enjoying the warmth of the sun and smelling the earth. This afforded him the ability to take short breaks every hundred feet while focusing on the environment. She showed him how to pay attention to each of those senses while deep breathing and focusing on the present moment. This technique enabled him to slowly increase his distance, and his connection to the universe broadened in step with his mindful walks. He was able to recover and go home with a new attitude. He said he would continue with the mindful walks, because they gave him great peace.

19

Vignettes–Real-Life Examples:
Guided Meditations

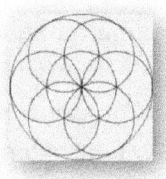

You need not wrestle for your good. Your good flows to you most easily when you are relaxed, open, and trusting.

~ALAN COHEN

Guided meditations are powerful in bringing back positive memories on many levels. The topics are endless. Some examples include awareness of breath, feelings and emotions, relaxation, and positive memories of beloved sacred spaces. Eliciting favorite memories of a sacred place from a patient or resident and walking that person into it can be a very spiritual experience. Creating impromptu guided meditations specific to the patient is powerful. In addition, there are many general guided meditation recordings out there that you can find on the Internet.

- W.S., a thirty-seven-year-old male, ordered by the court in lieu of prison to participate in a recovery program in a state-of-the-art, all-men's homeless shelter that had recovery and dual-diagnosis programs (men who had a psych diagnosis and also had a substance abuse diagnosis).

This was a pilot program that incorporated occupational therapy into the recovery program to teach life skills and run the dual-diagnosis program. This was a ninety-day mandatory program for W.S., who was in denial of his addiction even though he had very few teeth and had alienated his entire family with his behaviors. W.S. was angry and displayed many angry outbursts. He was at risk for being removed from the program, which meant he would be going back to jail. The OT began working with him on his socialization skills, and his inability to mix with the other men, whom he expressed were "beneath him." W.S. expressed feelings of hopelessness, and stated that he felt very alone in the world. W.S. projected a very tough exterior, often bragging about being the tough guy in his town. He used his anger to intimidate others. The OT introduced W.S. to guided meditations, first by asking for a fond memory of place. He responded, "I used to sit on the beach and watch the waves go in and out. This always got me back to normal." The OT took W.S. to a private and comfortable space.

Begin by sitting comfortably and relaxed. Picture yourself sitting on the beach with your eyes closed. You are completely comfortable, in loose clothing, in a pleasant position. Focus on your breath—slow and steady, in and out. Pay attention to the seagulls making their screeching noises as they fly over you and around you. Listen to the waves as they crash against rock and sand. Hear the children in the distance playing and laughing. Feel the warm and sunny salt air breeze across your body. You can taste the salt air as you breathe in through your mouth. Put your hands in the sand and feel the tiny grains between your fingers. Be there completely. While you are relaxed and feeling all your senses come alive with awareness, note the powder-blue sky and the clouds dreamily floating across the horizon above you. The waves are crashing with salty licks on the rocks and as they expand across the surface of the sand. You are at once at peace and calm. Sit here for a while and be there. Breathe in and out slowly. Be with your breath. This is where you need to go when you are feeling anger and anxiety.

The OT created a recording of this guided meditation that W.S. could listen to any time he felt anxiety or anger. W.S. stated he would try it. After a few weeks, W.S. continued to use this meditation and was able to stay in the program. By having a meditation that he could use any time he felt anxiety, he was able to overcome some of his anger issues and really focus on the recovery program. He was able to graduate and avoid jail.

- T.Y. was a sixty-one-year-old male admitted to the SNF; status: post–hip fracture due to a motor vehicle accident (MVA); and post–total hip replacement (THR). He also had multiple abrasions and a pretty severe laceration to his face, which required thirty-seven stitches. He lived alone but supported a daughter and ex-wife. T.Y. was self-employed as a framing contractor and had high anxiety about being able to return to work as soon as possible. He also reported being an avid hiker and nature lover. T.Y. had the daily habit during therapy of constantly complaining about his situation and blaming the MVA on the other driver. He was so highly focused on blame and the pending lawsuit he was planning to initiate that every time he spoke about it, his voice became louder, and he became agitated and angry all over again. It was disturbing the other patients in the gym and scaring some of them. The OT approached T.Y. to see if he would be open to a guided meditation experience, and he was agreeable. The OT and the patient went to a private area, and she prepared him by doing some relaxation techniques beginning with him sitting quietly in a comfortable position.

Close your eyes and think about each muscle, and deeply relax each one beginning in your feet. Then progress slowly up your body through the top of your head. Breathe through your nose, and on the inhale say the word peace *in your mind; and on the exhale say the word* trust. *Repeat* peace *and* trust *as you inhale and exhale.*

Now, imagine a time in your life when you were feeling really good. Where were you? Picture that memory and remember the place, and re-create the peaceful feeling you had. Remember how you felt then—your body was in excellent health, and you were at the top of your game, in peak condition. Breathe in the memory now. Your brain does not know the difference between then and now. Let all your cells and the fiber of your being re-experience this feeling of wellness. Notice that the feeling spreads across your body. It knows how to heal. Tell your body you know it knows what to do and that you will support this healing with your mind as well. With your healing thoughts and your inner knowing that your body knows how to heal itself, you begin to trust the process. You have watched your body heal itself throughout your life—scrapes, bruises, shaving cuts, and childhood traumas. You remember this now. Like the acorn that grows into a tree, you don't have to tell it what to do. It already knows. Focus on the knowledge that this, too, shall pass. You will heal. Everything will be OK. Keep the peaceful thoughts, and trust this process. Use this time to focus on peace and trust. Remember to breathe in and out the words peace *and* trust. *Focus your thoughts on this positive process. What you focus on in your thoughts tends to manifest in your reality, so keep a mindful watch on your thought process. Now take your time and be grateful that your body supports you. Let yourself gradually come back to the room, and let this wellness memory stay with you.*

T.Y. enjoyed this guided meditation. It became one of many. It also brought the OT and patient into a deeper connection beyond rapport, through deep listening. The OT approached this patient without judgment and with full acceptance. The therapist used this guided meditation to emphasize the positive and show a way to help the body heal by letting go of the resistance (complaining and being angry over and over about the same issue), emphasizing the focus on healing, and training the mind toward positive thoughts. This approach promoted a good outcome because the patient was guided to refocus his energy into healing in a nonconfrontational way and was able to change his behavior. He was able to go home much sooner than planned and had a good attitude at discharge.

20

Vignettes–Real-Life Examples:
Music

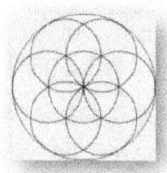

*"Ah, music," he said, wiping his eyes. "A magic beyond all
we do here!"*

~J. K. ROWLING, *HARRY POTTER AND THE SORCERER'S STONE*
(HARRY POTTER #1)

Music is the language of the soul and affords a deep connection through memory, time, and space. Certain music can bring back childhood memories, happy memories and sad memories, memories of place and times. Neuroscience tells us that the part of the brain that controls music appreciation is damaged last in the progression of dementia. Music can bridge emotions and memories and can bring even late-stage dementia patients back to life, even if for a short time of joy and peace.

- In a SNF with a locked dementia unit, the OT planned a rhythm group in the common area of the dementia unit. Residents had been in the facility on average for one to two years, and displayed moderate to late dementia symptoms. Instruments brought to the group included a few hand drums, maracas, finger bells, tambourines, and tom-toms. There were ten people in the room, and the rehab aide handed out instruments to each resident, and along with the OT demonstrated each instrument. One patient, M.M., a nonverbal resident, refused to take an instrument but remained in the room. The OT started out with a simple "heartbeat" of the hand drum and spoke about a baby's heartbeat. The rehab aide was able to assist residents in playing each instrument. It didn't take long for the residents to begin making sound, each with their own instrument, following the beat of the OT's drum as she shifted to a regular, steady beat. She shifted the beats and tempo. At first the sounds were totally unsynchronized, but residents soon fell into the rhythm with each of the different instruments. Each time she shifted the tempo and type of beat, residents soon followed. It was amazing to hear and see how the residents were able to follow the beats in a rhythmic and primal way. Residents seemed to come to life with each beat. You could see the connection and recognition that the residents were making to the primal beats. They were able to follow the OT in sync. M.M. began to clap her hands, alternating from top to bottom, over then under, right and left. Then she began to hum an old Southern gospel song with her hands clapping in sync with the group. This resident had not spoken in over a year, and yet she was singing and humming to the beat of the drum and clapping her hands rhythmically.

The OT scheduled the rhythm group every Friday. This was such a successful group that family members began attending as well as other staff. The group took on a life of its own. The connection and joy was evident and even if momentary, was considered a very effective and worthwhile event.

- T.F., an eighty-two-year-old male with moderate dementia, was a long-term care (LTC) resident in the SNF. He had become increasingly nonparticipatory, spoke very little, and sat in his wheelchair with his head on his padded lap tray much of the time. The patient was well known to the OT, and the OT was concerned about his more recent lack of engagement as she noted seeing him in the halls.

So she decided to ask his family what kind of music he liked. The family indicated he was a jazz fan in his younger years and gave some examples of his favorite musicians. The OT went to a thrift store that weekend and found some old CDs of jazz musicians of the 1940s and 1950s. She facilitated a therapy group titled "Music Appreciation," and invited several residents at varying stages of dementia, mild to moderate, including T.F. When she turned on the music, T.F. became aware, and as if he had awoken from a long nap, raised his head off the lap table and began humming to the music, swaying his head left and right, eyes closed. It was as if he became alive again. He listened intently and soon had tears of joy running down his cheeks. The group was asked to discuss their experience of the music. The higher-level residents were able to talk about the evoked memories the music inspired in them. Even T.F. was able to convey his emotion at the memories, and although he was not able to articulate it very well in descriptive words, the joy was evident in his facial expression. The music appreciation group was a shared experience, and the group became a weekly event. T.F.'s family gave him a CD player, and they assisted him by playing several CDs in his room. The nursing staff played his music for him as well. His whole demeanor changed. He was able to enjoy the music even as the dementia progressed, until he passed away from a myocardial infarction later that year.

21

Vignettes–Real-Life Examples: Aromatherapy

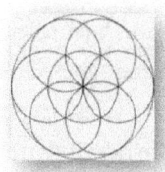

At no other time (than autumn) does the earth let itself be inhaled in one smell, the ripe earth; in a smell that is in no way inferior to the smell of the sea, bitter where it borders on taste, and more honeysweet where you feel it touching the first sounds. Containing depth within itself, darkness, something of the grave almost.

~RAINER MARIA RILKE, *LETTERS ON CÉZANNE*

Aromatherapy can be a powerful and safe intervention to relieve stress, pain, and anxiety, and increase calm and focus. It is also a great alternative to antipsychotics use in the SNF setting with patients diagnosed with dementia.

- T.T. was a sixty-one-year-old female LTC resident in the SNF within a dementia unit. She had moderate dementia and had been recovering from a urinary tract infection (UTI) and was weak from her five-day hospital stay. She also had chronic obstructive pulmonary disease (COPD) but did not require continuous oxygen therapy. The OT's goals for T.T. were for self-feeding, to return to her prior level of function (PLOF), stand-by assist (SBA) and distant supervision; and basic grooming activities with SBA, with setup and occasional verbal cues to stay on task. Since returning from the hospital, T.T. had been experiencing sundowning. The OT was asked to assess for environmental interventions to help the nursing staff with the new-onset sundowning behaviors. The OT had an essential oil compound mix for calming and anxiety that consisted of geranium, lavender, and bergamot in a sweet almond carrier oil. The OT clocked in later several days in a row so she could stay down in the dementia unit and train the nursing staff on the use of aromatherapy in the evenings. When T.T. became agitated, she put a few drops on a cotton ball and put the cotton ball next to T.T. That did calm her down. The next day she added a few drops of the mixture to unscented lotion and applied it topically to T.T.'s face and arms. She stayed long enough to see if there would be a reaction to the application, and there was not. T.T. continued to have less agitation. After a week of applying the lotion to T.T. with the aromatherapy essential oils mixture, the anxiety and agitation subsided altogether.

The facility's medical director commended the OT for this environmental adaptation, acknowledged the benefit and use of aromatherapy with cotton balls, and of the lotion mixed with the essential oils, which when indicated, became a normal course in the dementia unit.

22

Vignettes–Real-Life Examples:
Pet Therapy

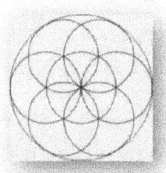

Until one has loved an animal, a part of one's soul remains
unawakened.

~ANATOLE FRANCE

Pet therapy provides patients, residents, or clients comfort and aids in recovery from many medical diagnoses. Pets bring unconditional love, elicit memories of long-ago beloved pets, and increase social interaction while reducing a sense of isolation and disconnection.

- M.M., a fifty-three-year-old male veteran, out of the military for two years, admitted to a SNF after being hit by a car, sustaining a hip fracture; status: post- surgery with an open reduction internal fixation (ORIF), which involves the use of plates and screws or a intramedullary rod to stabilize the bone. M.M. showed signs and symptoms of depression, isolating himself, refusing to come to therapy, and being belligerent to staff. The pain was poorly controlled due to his refusal of medications. The OT was very concerned and worked on establishing rapport with M.M. In her interaction with M.M., the OT learned he had a Dutch-German shepherd mix named Duke (after John Wayne) that had performed in Afghanistan as a bomb-sniffing dog at Combat Outpost Ahmad Khan (AK) in Kandahar Province. M.M. was his last handler in the war. M.M. explained that Duke and he had a very special bond and shared a spiritual connection. M.M. was able to adopt Duke upon his discharge because he was the last handler and Duke was also being retired after ten years of service.

Duke was staying with M.M.'s sister while he was an inpatient at the SNF. The OT called the sister and inquired about the dog. The SNF had many rules about visiting animals, and the OT had to ask the sister to produce Duke's shot records and license, and sign a statement that the dog did not have a history of biting. Then the facility issued him a name tag like all the staff wore. The OT arranged for a surprise visit from Duke, timed appropriately while M.M. was scheduled to be in the therapy gym. M.M. was having a bad day and refused to come to the gym at the selected time. The OT convinced him to come eventually while other patients were in the gym having a group session. Duke came in, and when he saw M.M. in his wheelchair, he was so excited that he ran over to him, licked him, and jumped on him. M.M. had tears of joy running down his cheeks at the reunion. In fact, there wasn't a dry eye in the room for the joy of witnessing this lovely event.

M.M.'s mood lightened thereafter, and Duke became a regular visitor, bringing joy to M.M. and the staff and other patients as well. M.M. began participating in therapy, and Duke became part of therapy, with M.M. playing fetch with Duke with the purpose of "exercising his dog."

After witnessing the powerful effect of this pet therapy on the patient and the entire staff, the facility administrator gave permission for the facility to reach out to the local community and schedule regular visits from local rescue animals. One volunteer brought rabbits in their cages and took them around to the gym and patients' rooms.

Another volunteer brought in her rescue pugs. Pet therapy became a regular and welcomed event.

23

Vignettes–Real-Life Examples: Gardening

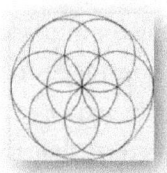

I love spring anywhere, but if I could choose I would always greet it in a garden.

-RUTH STOUT

Gardening is an age-old pastime familiar to most people. It can bring a sense of connection to the earth, be a perfect setting for mindfulness, and provide a perfect opportunity for a group experience.

- T.W., a sixty-five-year-old LTC patient in a SNF with a diagnosis of multiple sclerosis (MS), disclosed that her favorite pastime when she lived at home was to work in the garden and "grow things." The OT thought this would be a great part of therapy and would facilitate healing time in the fresh air, and work on upper body strength and coordination; she also thought it would be good for T.W.'s spiritual reconnection. The OT asked the administrator if she and T.W. could clean up in the courtyard garden and plant some flowers. The administrator agreed. T.W. insisted on sweeping the courtyard from her wheelchair in anticipation of the activity. T.W. was currently in remission from MS, and although she normally used a wheelchair, she could walk short distances. The OT was able to obtain some pots, potting soil, and seeds. T.W. was able to sit at the picnic table in her wheelchair in the courtyard and work on her fine motor coordination, range of motion, and strength in her upper body through lifting the small pots, adding the potting soil, and handling the seeds. The OT was also able to purchase a small six-pack of tulips that T.W. was able to transplant into some pots to arrange around the courtyard. This activity was so enjoyable to T.W. that she came out every day on her own to monitor the plants and water them. As they began to grow, her spiritual well-being continued to grow as well. T.W. exclaimed, "I feel more content than I have in a very long time."

The administrator agreed that the gardening activity was a worthy activity to pursue further. He had four large, raised garden containers built by the maintenance man, who was able to install a crank to adjust the height of the beds, like a high/low table. This was a perfect therapy spot and destination because it became the talk of the facility. Physical therapists (PTs) were able to have patients stand at the garden table for endurance while they planted and worked the garden. OTs were able to also stand patients or have them seated in their wheelchairs or a regular chair for endurance while the patients weeded, planted, or watered. This activity was a catalyst for spiritual reconnection for everyone involved, including the therapists. The discussions with patients as a group were also very valuable in sharing the experience, memories that the activity brought back, and the mindfulness and spiritual connections to the earth.

24

Vignettes–Real-Life Examples: Creativity

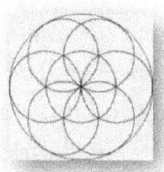

Listening is a magnetic and strange thing, a creative force. The friends who listen to us are the ones we move toward. When we are listened to, it creates us, makes us unfold and expand.

~Shel Silverstein

Creativity is a direct link to Spirit, whether it is through music, art, dance, writing, or other avenues. Creative therapy is a powerful tool to help dissolve the perception of disconnection and help patients and clients to bring out feelings of empowerment and recognize their inherent value to the whole. Think outside the box for creative therapy in any occupational therapy setting. We only need to be creative ourselves to establish some valuable ideas for therapy in each unique setting.

- The OT wanted to form a creativity group with residents in a "personal care home" for persons with a psychological (psych) diagnosis, a voluntary in-patient program that was funded by the state. Below is a description of the setting:

- There were twenty-five females and twenty-seven males in the personal care home, with gender-separate sleeping accommodations at opposite ends of the building with a common area to mingle and have social interaction. Common diagnoses in this setting were borderline personality disorder, schizophrenia, schizoaffective disorder, bipolar disorder, and posttraumatic stress disorder. Residents in this care home were unable to function independently on the outside and voluntarily entered this program. The main focus of the program was to teach life skills with a goal of being able to go back out to an independent setting if possible. There was a nurse at all times in both the female and male sections, and they dispersed the medications for all residents. Part of the condition of the program was to consistently take the prescribed medications. In the world of psych treatment, taking the meds regularly is integral to success. (The common problem on the outside for people with psych diagnoses is they do not stay on their meds, and the cycle of symptoms exacerbates while out in the community.)

The OT decided to start with a women's creativity group, beginning with journal writing as an avenue for self-discovery and connection to the spiritual higher self. There had been much arguing in the women's section, fighting over what to watch on the only TV, and other personal bickering and incidents of unwanted and inappropriate male attention. The goal of the group was to increase the perception of spiritual connection, self-esteem, and self-discovery through writing, by identifying and exploring residents' feelings, increasing cohesion in the group, and creating a sense of personal empowerment and self-worth. The format was a five-week biweekly meeting with "topic" discussion first, then required daily entries in the journal, even if just one sentence (sometimes it was a challenge to get consistent participation with residents in this setting), then follow-up discussion at the next meeting on the previous topic, and the introduction and brief discussion of the new topic. Participation and attendance was required in order to stay in the group. The OT had a good rapport with these residents, and they wanted to participate. Topics for each group meeting and assigned journal topics included the following:

1. Prayer
2. Knowing your value
3. Getting along with your neighbors
4. Finding the *Big* Me (the golden rule)
5. Five ways to nurture the self
6. Creating self-love in your life
7. Keeping our bodies private
8. How to say no and mean it (no means no) (setting boundaries is good!)
9. Happiness
10. Friendship

The seven women who joined the group were between twenty-seven and forty-nine years old, and the diagnoses in the group included schizophrenia, schizoaffective disorder, bipolar disorder, and borderline personality disorder. There was a wide range of levels of lower-end emotional intelligence, and the completed educational level of the group was on average tenth grade. The writing-level ability was variable, but that was not the focus—it was on the content and sharing ideas presented. The OT supplied the group of seven females with pens and composition books. After the group was established and residents became comfortable, some of the discussion topics elicited further questions, discussion, solutions, conclusions, and stories throughout the five-week course:

- We are all connected, so if we hurt one person, we hurt ourselves.

- We are all children of Spirit, so we all have equal love—no one is better or worse than anyone else.
- What does it mean to respect another's space?
- How can we demonstrate that respect?
- What is a way that we can share the TV? Take turns being able to choose the programs?
- What does it mean to be the bigger person (and walk away instead of arguing)?
- Five ways to nurture ourselves—the group decided on talking to God (prayer); having alone time to think (silent contemplation); being happy with where we are (gratitude); thinking about now instead of the past or worrying about tomorrow (mindfulness); and being kind to others (compassion for others).
- We have to love ourselves in order to love others.
- We only share our bodies in private and only if we want to.
- It is OK to say no and set boundaries with others.
- Happiness is what we think about, so stay happy in our thinking.
- Having friends is the spice of life.

This group was unusually successful for this setting because the women consistently attended. Evidence of more cooperation led to a more peaceful overall atmosphere in the care home, and the group was adopted as a regular ongoing group. The OT also started a similar men's group.

- The next group established in the personal care home became a women's art group on Mondays and Wednesdays. Art supplies were limited due to funding, so the first idea was doing collages with donated magazines. The goal of the group was to pick a theme and have the women go through the magazines and cut and paste words and images into a collage. The first theme was "calming." The instructions were to find images you find soothing and calming, and cut and paste them onto the paper into a collage. During the group the OT played very soothing instrumental music. The result was beautiful collages from each and every one of them. The point of the art project was to introduce them to identifying their calming triggers and to find images that convey calm for them, and to be able to hang the collage in their rooms and to seek the collage as a calming tool when they began feeling anxious. It was a very positive experience and a positive tool for them.

Other art ideas and themes that were implemented in the art group include finger painting; drawing in the dark (to free the mind from judging); painting images or doing collages of our good traits; making art out of our fingerprints; and decorating shoe boxes for a "prayer box" and adding a slit at the top. Residents could put pieces of paper with messages of their deepest prayers for Spirit. It could also be used as a "gratitude box."

• Another men and women's joint group in the personal care home was learning a simple line dance together. It was a fun and social exercise to create body, mind, and spiritual health; explore social interaction without intimate touching; introduce a fun way to set boundaries; decrease inhibitions and self-consciousness in participating in dance; and establish a fun interaction to add cohesion and cooperation in the group. Participants loved this group! It also established a calming atmosphere in the home and brought the residents together in camaraderie.

25

Vignettes–Real-Life Examples: Humor

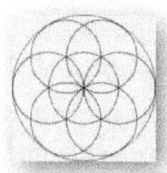

Before you criticize someone, you should walk a mile in their shoes. That way, when you criticize them, you're a mile away and you have their shoes.

~JACK HANDEY

Laughter is the best medicine. It is free and available to anyone who has the right mind-set. It is so good to facilitate laughter in a health-care setting. It lifts people up, and sharing the laughter becomes contagious. Laughter is a universal language and a fast way to share.

- R.T., a sixty-eight-year-old male LTC resident of the SNF, with a diagnosis of chronic obstructive pulmonary disease (COPD), had expressed feelings of sadness during an occupational therapy treatment one day, saying that his children were too far away and could not visit him (they both lived in two different states and had to fly to come to the facility for a visit). The OT arranged a weekly Skype visit with each of the two daughters on the facility computer in a family conference room. During one of the visits, the OT noticed that R.T. loved to tell his daughters jokes. He would tell the same jokes to both daughters on separate occasions, and he'd get the biggest laugh of all in the telling. It was evident that this was how he related to his children over a lifetime. The OT asked R.T. if he would bring his best joke to the therapy gym the next day. He told the joke with delight and had all the other patients in the gym laughing. This gave him a great sense of pleasure. He began to supply a new joke every day to all the patients in the gym. The OT decided to have a weekly Friday joke-fest and invited all the patients to come prepared with their best jokes. This became a regular happening and was called Thank God it's Friday (TGIF)-Joke Friday. All patients were asked to supply a joke, like having a secret password, to gain entrance into the gym. Even the staff had to have the secret password, a joke, to gain entrance. The majority of staff and patients who were able participated in good faith. As patients came and went, the TGIF-Joke Friday evolved, and the OT began showing short episodes of *The Three Stooges*, followed by discussions about humor and the memories evoked, and the place of humor in getting well. The facility began showing comedy movies on Fridays as well to join in the fun. TGIF-Joke Fridays was a hit all around and met the needs of patients and staff in creating the shared experience of humor and the healing it fostered in mind, body, and spirit.

26

Sacred Roots and Wings

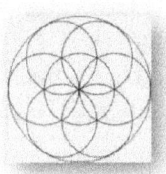

*It is one of the most beautiful compensations of this life that no
man can sincerely try to help another without helping himself...
Serve and thou shall be served.*

~RALPH WALDO EMERSON

Occupational therapy practitioners are indeed in a unique position to change
the world, one patient, one family, one community, one country, and one universe at a time. Spiritual integration and occupational therapy are naturally
intertwined because we share the same language and see through the same
lens. We practice self-compassion through gratitude, meditation, mindfulness, music, creativity, and humor, and whatever brings peace to life...on a
daily basis.

We anchor our own sacred roots and wings and foster roots and wings
in others, with reverence for all wisdom, all faiths, all spiritual paths, all
religions, and agnostic and atheist pathways in our sacred compassion for
others. We are brave and awake, and bring our authentic and whole heart-
self to all our interactions by living consciously. We set our intentions and
follow the Light. We share rapport, listen deeply, form sacred connections,

and take sacred actions. We share our stories to help one another be all that we can be. We bring our sacredness to the therapeutic use of self in all our treatment.

There is a long and beautiful history of the evolution of the essence of spirituality, drawn on the ancient masters: The progressive knowledge that spiritual thinkers built and expanded upon in the nineteenth and twentieth centuries is now expanding the essence of spirituality exponentially in the twenty-first century. People are hungry for more—more authentic connection, more belonging, more love and acceptance—and are demanding change in current religious traditions. People are reaching out to New Thought thinkers, teachers, and ideals, which are becoming increasingly mainstream, integrating the philosophy into their spiritual belief system and at times complementing their religious beliefs. A golden thread of truth spins through the tapestry of all religions and all spiritual paths to Truth: the essence of spirituality is *connection*. Follow the cosmic Wi-Fi, where the connection is absolute.

Spiritual connection is vital to health and wellness in mind, body, and spirit to everyone, *regardless of their awareness*. The world is in a state of chaos because of a huge universal lack of awareness of our inherent cosmic connection, which has brought on a new thought "revolution." We have to change our approach to life. Albert Einstein said, "Insanity is doing the same thing over and over and expecting different results." We cannot bring change to the world doing everything the same way we always have. We have to change our thinking and our culture of thought. Remember the experience of Frankl in the Nazi concentration camps, who later concluded that survival is based on strength derived from purpose and discovering the meaning in one's life and experience.

We are all one and just walking one another home. We all belong to one another. One person's perceived disconnection impacts us all, either directly or indirectly. One person's disconnection is every person's disconnection. One person's connection is every person's connection. Doing what makes us come alive is what the world needs—more people who have come alive. Helping others connect is the first step in their healing…and helps us to come alive. It is always the journey, not the destination—right here, right now, this moment.

Understanding how to utilize the resources and tools to foster a sense of spiritual connection and reconnection within occupational therapy treatment and adjunct therapeutic activities will help us all succeed in creating a better world, by raising the planetary vibration one person at a time and helping more and more people to remember who they are, fostering healing in mind, body, and spirit.

Rumi said, "The Universe and the light of the world shines through me."

27

Resources/Toolkit

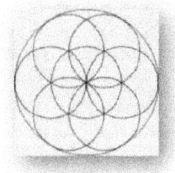

God has no religion.

~Gandhi

Spirituality
Web and E-mail
revsandywest@live.com
http://consciousnesshealing.net/
http://freedomthroughchoice.org/ (Freedom through Choice Foundation)
http://krystalsinger.com/
http://lifepurposehelp.com/
http://spiritualityandhealth.com/
http://www.onenessusa.org/index.php/oneness/oneness-university.html
http://emersoninstitute.edu/

Twitter
@aquariflame

Facebook

Sacred Roots and Wings, Krystal Singer, Life Purpose Help, Positive Living Center

YouTube
2SistersChat
Positive Living Center

TV
Super Soul Sunday on OWN

Gratitude
Any of the spirituality resources can be of help on gratitude.

Aromatherapy
http://www.mydoterra.com/mygarden/
https://www.aromaticscience.com/
https://www.auracacia.com/
http://www.lotionlady.com/
http://living-essential-oils.com/
https://www.youngliving.org/oils4wellness

Gardening
http://www.gardensall.com/?s=55+gal+drum+raised+beds
　　You can reach out to local churches or the community to see if they have access to building a raised garden for the community skilled nursing facility.
http://www.thisoldhouse.com/toh/m/video/0,,20788577,00.html
　　Google Lowes and Home Depot for how to build a raised garden for wheelchair access. There are YouTube videos on this as well.

Reach out to your local garden club for volunteer lectures and garden guidance.

Meditation

https://chopracentermeditation.com/

Deepak Chopra and Oprah Winfrey offer a free twenty-one-day meditation series on a different topic:

http://www.oprah.com/oprahs-lifeclass/Register-Now-for-the-21-Day-Meditation-Challenge

YouTube has many guided meditations.

Search Amazon.com for guided meditation DVDs and CDs.

Music

Highly recommended documentary: *Alive Inside: A Story of Music and Memory,* based on the work of Dan Cohen, MSW, and directed by Michael Rossato-Bennett. It will completely change your perspective in treating patients with dementia.

All books by Christine Stevens, MSW, MT-BC (see references)

Pet Therapy

Contact and network in your community with rescue groups and resources.

Humor

Most local libraries have a huge selection of videos and DVDs for comedies geared toward the era you are looking for. Also live streaming and YouTube have much available. For example:

Buster Keaton movies from the 1920s to the 1950s
The Three Stooges

Abbott & Costello shows (I love "Who's on First")
Carol Burnett shows (My favorite is the "Dentist Skit" with Tim Conway and Harvey Korman)
The Smothers brothers
The Marx brothers

References

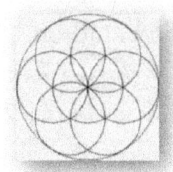

Aldridge, David. "Spirituality, Hope and Music Therapy in Palliative Care." *The Arts in Psychotherapy* 22, no. 2 (1995): 103–109.

American Occupational Therapy Association. "Scope of Practice." *American Journal of Occupational Therapy* 58, no. 6 (2004): 673.

American Occupational Therapy Association. *Occupational Therapy Practice Framework: Domain & Process.* 3rd ed. Bethesda, MD: American Occupational Therapy Association, 2014.

Ballard, Clive G., John T. O'Brien, Katherine Reichelt, and Elaine Perry. "Aromatherapy as a Safe and Effective Treatment for the Management of Agitation in Severe Dementia: The Results of a Double-Blind, Placebo-Controlled Trial." *Journal of Clinical Psychiatry* 63, no. 7 (2002): 553–558.

Blumberg, Antonia. "Rabbi Denise Eger to Become First Openly Gay President of the Central Conference of American Rabbis." *Huffingtonpost. com*, March 13, 2015. http://www.huffingtonpost.com/2015/03/13/rabbi-denise-eger-president-ccar_n_6848156.html.

Buddha Groove, http://www.buddhagroove.com/

Buddha Groove. "10 Thoughts on Spirituality." www.buddhagroove.com/10-thoughts-on-spirituality/.

Buddha Groove. "Meditation in Different Traditions." http://www.buddhagroove.com/meditation-in-different-traditions/.

Brown, Brené. *Daring Greatly.* New York: Gotham Books, 2012.

Campbell, Joseph. *The Hero with a Thousand Faces.* Princeton, NJ: Princeton University Press, 1949.

Chopra, Deepak. "3 Essential Practices for Gratitude." *Spirituality & Health,* 2015. http://spiritualityhealth.com/articles/3-essential-practices-gratitude.

Dalai Lama and Howard Cutler. *The Art of Happiness: A Handbook for Living.* New York: Riverhead Books, 1998.

Dissanayake, Ellen. *Conversations before the End of Time.* Edited by Suzi Gablick London: Thames and Hudson, 1995.

Dyer, Wayne. *Change Your Thoughts—Change Your Life: Living the Wisdom of the Tao.* Carlsbad, CA: Hay House, 2007. Emerson Institute, http://emersoninstitute.edu

EnergyandVibration.com. "Vibrational Energy Medicine Principles." January 2, 2013. http://energyandvibration.com/energymedicine.htm.

Fick, Katherine M. "The Influence of an Animal on Social Interactions of Nursing Home Residents in a Group Setting." *American Journal of Occupational Therapy* 47, no. 6 (1993): 529-534

Gawande, Atul. *Being Mortal: Medicine and What Matters in the End.* New York: Metropolitan Books, 2014.

Haupt, Jennifer. "Channeling Depression into a Powerful Tool for Creativity." 2015. http://spiritualityandhealth.com/articles/channeling-depression-powerful-tool-creativity.

Higginbotham, Melissa. "Voicing the Sound Eternal." PhD diss., Emerson Theological Institute, 2014.

Hooper, B., and W. Wood. "The Philosophy of Occupational Therapy: A Framework for Practice." In *Willard and Spackman's Occupational Therapy,* 12th ed. Edited by B. A. Boyt Schell, G. Gillen, and M. Scaffa. Philadelphia: Lippincott Williams & Wilkins, 2014.

Kabat-Zinn, Jon. *Full Catastrophe Living: Using the Wisdom of Your Body and Mind to Face Stress, Pain, and Illness.* New York: Dell Publishing, 1990.

King, Brian E. "Humor, Laughter, and Health." Course sponsored by the Institute for Brain Potential, Fresno, CA, 2014.

Kuruvilla, Carol. "3 Ways Pope Francis Delighted and Disappointed Us at the Same Time." *Huffingtonpost.com*, March 13, 2015. http://www.huffingtonpost. com/2015/03/13/pope-francis-2-year-anniversary_n_6859224.html.

Loken, Camillo. "Is Everything Energy?" 2015. http://www.one-mind-one-energy.com/energy.htm.

Mayo Clinic. "Pet Therapy: Man's Best Friend as Healer: Animal-Assisted Therapy Can Help Healing and Lessen Depression and Fatigue." 2015. http://www.mayoclinic.org/healthy-lifestyle/consumer-health/in-depth/pet-therapy/art-20046342.

Meulman, Monika. "Essential Oils in the Autistic Classroom—Pilot Study." 2009. http://healingmuse.com/toronto/inspired-healing/essential-oils-in-the-autistic-classroom-pilot-study/.

Music & Memory Certification Program, http://www.musicandmemory.org/

Osbon, Diane K. *Reflections on the Art of Living: A Joseph Campbell Companion.* New York: HarperCollins, 1991. Oneness University, http://onenessuniversity. org

Padilla, Rene. "Effectiveness of Environment-Based Interventions for People with Alzheimer's Disease and Related Dementia." *American Journal of Occupational Therapy* 65 (2011): 514–522.

Paintner, Christine Valters. "The Relationship between Spirituality and Artistic Expression: Cultivating the Capacity for Imagining." *Spirituality in Higher Education Newsletter* 3, no. 2 (2007).

Park, H., and VanLeit, B. "The Meaning of Gardening for Adults with Developmental Disabilities." *AOTA*, Special Interest Section Quarterly, 36, (1), 1-3 March 2012

Puchalski, C., Ferrell, B., Virani, R., Otis-Green, S., Baird, P., J. Bull, J., Chochinov, H., Handzo, G., Nelson-Becker, H., Prince-Paul, M., Pugliese, K., and Sulmasy, D, 2009. "Improving the Quality of Spiritual Care as a Dimension of Palliative Care: The Report of the Consensus Conference." *Journal of Palliative Medicine* 12 (2009): 885-904.

Punwar, A. J., and Peloquin, S. M. . *Occupational Therapy Principles and Practice.* 3rd ed. Philadelphia: Lippincott Williams and Wilkins, 2000.

"Ralph Waldo Emerson." http://transcendentalism-legacy.tamu.edu/authors/emerson/.

Stevens, Christine. *Music Medicine: The Science and Spirit of Healing Yourself with Sound.* Boulder, CO: Sounds True, 2012.

Science Daily, http://www.sciencedaily.com/

Tan, Chade-Meng. *Search Inside Yourself: The Unexpected Path to Achieving Success, Happiness (and World Peace).* New York: HarperCollins, 2012.

Thich Nhat Hanh. *Peace Is Every Step: The Path of Mindfulness in Everyday Life.* New York: Bantam Books, 1992.

———. *Happiness.* Berkeley, CA: Parallax Press, 2009.

Tolle, Eckhart. *The Power of Now.* Novato, CA: Namaste Publishing and New World Library, 1999.

———. *A New Earth: Awakening to Your Life's Purpose.* New York: Plume, 2005.

Tolles, Jim. "Spiritual Awakening Process: Spirituality and Humor: Finding Laughter in Your Life." 2012. http://www.spiritualawakeningprocess.com.

Troward, Thomas. "The Edinburgh Lectures on Mental Science." 1904. http://www.newthoughtlibrary.com.

Science of Mind Magazine, http://www.Scienceofmind.com

http://www.solitarius.org

http://www.spiritualityhealth.com

Welch, John. *Spiritual Pilgrims: Carl Jung and Teresa of Avila.* New York: Paulist Press, 1982.

Zisselman, M., Rovner, B., Shmuely, Y., Ferrie, P.. "A Pet Therapy Intervention with Geriatric Psychiatry Inpatients." *American Journal of Occupational Therapy* 50, no. 1 (1996): 47-51.

The Flower of Life
Where Math, Geometry, and Spirituality Meet

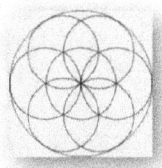

The Flower of Life is an ancient religious symbol of the sacred geometry, which contains a secret shape known as the Fruit of Life and represents ancient spiritual beliefs. It contains seven or more overlapping circles in which the center of each circle is on the circumference of up to six surrounding circles of the same diameter that hold many mathematical and geometrical laws. These laws represent the whole Universe. According to Drunvalo Melchizedek, author and teacher, the Flower of Life depicts aspects of encoded creation patterns for the fundamental forms of space and time, thought to act as a template from which all life springs.

The Flower of Life symbol can be found in all the major religions of the world. In Egypt, whose tradition many people believe is the source of all the monotheistic religions, the Flower of Life can be found in the ancient temple of Abydos. In Israel, it can be found in the ancient synagogues of the Galilee and in the Masada. The Flower of Life is found incised on roof beams of a ceiling dating from 1681 in Poland and thought to provide protection from lightning.

The Flower of Life is one of the strongest sacred geometric shapes in the world.

About the Author

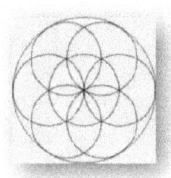

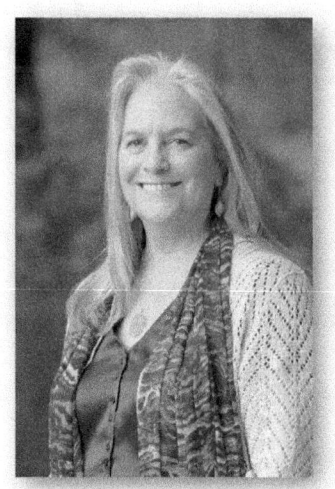

Laura Ayres Hayth holds a doctorate in spiritual studies from Emerson Theological Institute, a master's certificate in health-care corporate compliance from George Washington University, and a bachelor of science in occupational therapy from Eastern Kentucky University.

Laura has published many internal company articles throughout her career, including "Low Vision, Low Tech Solutions in the SNF Setting."

Laura is currently an area vice president in a large national therapy company, which contracts therapy in nursing homes, home health, and rehab agency (outpatient). She was recently appointed by Governor Jerry Brown to serve on the California Board of Occupational Therapy.

You can find her Facebook page at Sacred Roots and Wings, and web page at www.lauraayreshayth.com.

Laura lives near Yosemite, enjoys the peaceful mountain setting, loves the beach, and enjoys writing, painting, and living with her two cats, Honey and

Marilyn Monroe. She enjoys her connection with her two adult children, their spouses, and her grandson.

Laura is a certified Deeksha giver (Oneness Blessing). She enjoys the on-going and never-ending spiritual growth experience.